2009

Dim Mak Secrets
Pressure Points
Secrets of Fighting
and Self Defense   &
True Secrets of
Extreme Flexibility

A.Thomas Perhacs

A compilation of four powerful manuscripts on Dim Mak Training and Self-defense

Scientific Premium Company-USA
Velocity Group Publishing © Copyright 2009 All Rights Reserved

Preface

DISCLAIMER

Neither A. Thomas Perhacs nor Velocity Group Publishing assumes any responsibility for the use or misuse of the concepts, methods and strategies contained in this book. The reader is warned that the use of some or all of the techniques in this book may result in legal consequences, civil and/or criminal.

USE OF THIS BOOK IS DONE AT YOUR OWN RISK.

(Updated Version, July 2009)

When I first wrote the material in this book, I considered it to be quite a bit different than most of the other works I had seen on the market, and I wondered if I even wanted to publish the material. I did extensive research finding out how a lot of these things work through my own experiences and those of students, colleagues and friends I have met over the years. This book actually contains four (4) of my most popular manuscripts:

Dim Mak Secrets

Pressure Points

Secrets of Fighting and Self Defense

True Secrets of Extreme Flexibility

I believe the information in this manual is fresh and will allow you to begin to understand yet another facet of your dim mak training.

Most people, who have read this material have claimed they were some of the best books they have read and in fact answered a lot of their questions. I hope you will find it to be the same for you. Enjoy this book as the insights are interesting…to say the least.

Sifu Perhacs
Hamilton, New Jersey
July 2009

Table of Contents

Part IV

Part I:

Dim Mak Secrets

By Scientific Premium Company-USA

Published by Velocity Group Publishing

PO Box 9516 Hamilton, NJ 08650

© Copyright 2009 All Rights Reserved

The Deadly Secrets of Dim Mak Vital Point Striking

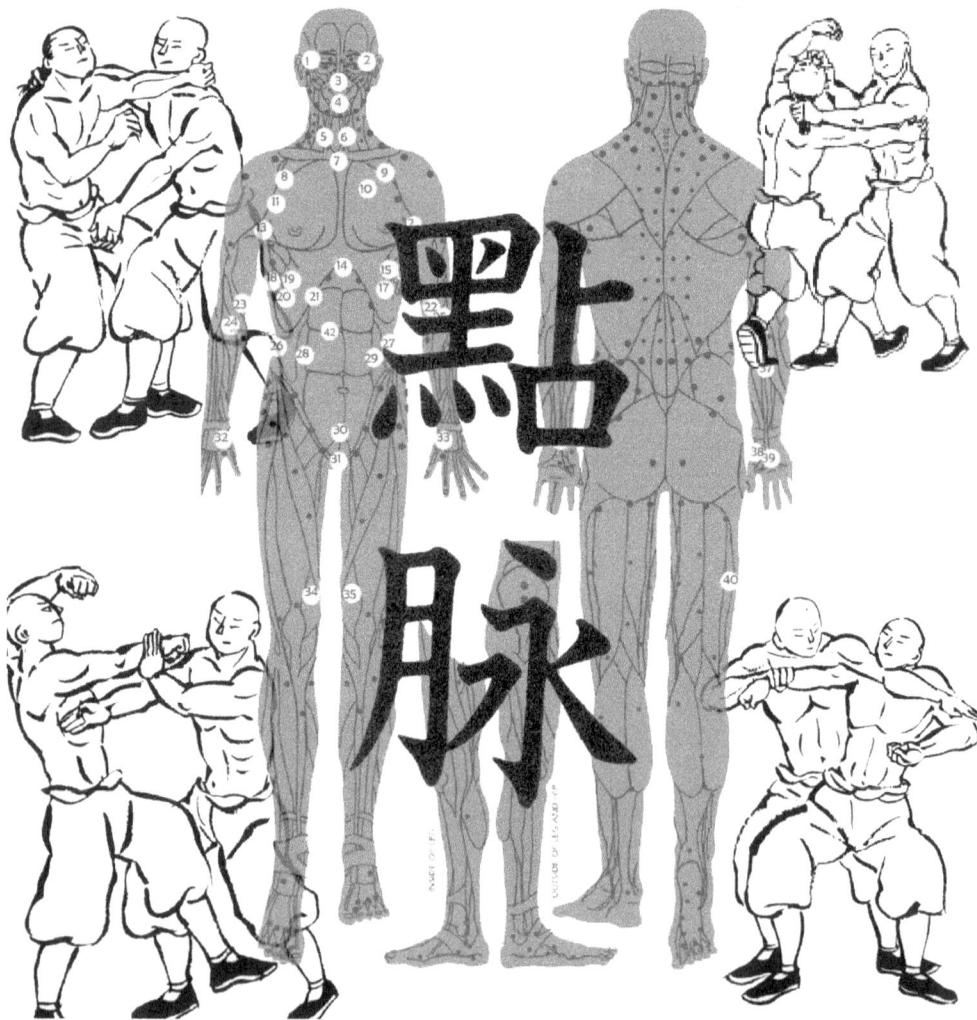

Introduction

Dim Mak is one of the most closely guarded secrets in the fighting world. Legends tell stories of the fabled "Death Touch". Some have even said that a Chinese Tong member killed Bruce Lee with a delayed "Death Touch". Of course a lot of what is taught about Dim Mak is conjecture at best.

What we want to do with this additional report on Dim Mak, is try and add some additional information for you on how to approach these techniques to add into your martial arts curriculum.

__Scientific Premium Company- USA makes the claim that the information described here are for information purposes only and we accept no responsibility for your use of these concepts to hurt, maim or intentionally or unintentionally end a life. It is with this caution that we suggest you get a qualified instructor to teach you in your area.__

The pressure and Dim Mak points that we are going to be discussing absolutely work and work very well. It is our belief that you can learn how to use Dim Mak striking methods without harming anyone if you are careful.

It will be your sole responsibility to use this information with the utmost care and sensitivity. **DO NOT TAKE THESE TECHNIQUES, CONCEPTS AND METHODS AND START STRIKING PEOPLE!**

Only use these points for the purpose of self- preservation or for healing.

Why Teach These Deadly Concepts?

One of the main reasons we have made this information available is so that you can have access to what was once a closely guarded secret. Many went to their deaths without knowing the knowledge you will learn with this.

The other reason we teach this, is because although we have packed a lot of information into this curriculum and, we have purposefully left out some elements in regards to some of the more lethal "Chi Striking" techniques. However, you may learn these from us personally by inquiring by email or phone. We will only teach those methods to the most ethical and reliable of people, and normally only in our closed system of training.

We consider these concepts as deadly as any other weapon you can use, so why not teach it to only responsible people? Anyone can buy a gun with malicious intent and use it in the wrong way against another person.

The real secret to these points is not the death that they can cause, but the health and life you can preserve by using these techniques correctly (See Pressure Points Booklet).

The other reason why we teach this type material, is because since 1980, we have been introducing cutting edge products like our Chi Power Plus and Pressure Points Courses. We taught thousands, the secrets of how to use their chi energy when everyone else teaching was behind closed doors. We continue that open door policy with this eye-opening course on how to use pressure points for Dim Mak Striking.

Levels of Dim Mak

There are several levels to the type of damage you can inflict with Dim Mak strikes and there are many factors in regards to how effective the strikes will be against an opponent. You really only have seconds to use these strikes, so it is imperative that you understand the importance of training with the strikes regularly, to get down where the different striking points are located.

Dim Mak as a striking system has been around for thousands of years and probably was known before it was ever recorded on paper. For martial arts purposes, almost every culture has an understanding of not only pressure points, but also the ability to use energy or chi with these Dim Mak Points.

Dim Mak is taken from the Chinese word for "Death Point Striking" and is considered by many as one of the highest levels in the martial arts. Most students never learned these methods until they were at the Black Belt or equivalent level (depending on the school and style). These structures were taught in China, but were transferred to other cultures such as Japanese and Korean. As mentioned before, almost all cultures have this understanding, but it is believed the Chinese were at the forefront.

Once you begin to absorb the information here, you will realize one thing and that is that this is a science that has some disagreements to it. We will be sharing with you several different points and striking methods. We will show these through our own chart (redman poster) and several others throughout this document.

Many of the points discussed in one chart may be different than those of another. Keep in mind that in order to understand the potency of this technology, Chinese doctors would strike these points on animals to insure that the strikes, in-fact worked as they thought they would.

These vital points were taught as part of an overall self defense curriculum at the time which included, Striking and Kicking methods; joint locks; chokes; take-downs; throws; hand and leg maneuvers; grappling; escapes; ground-work; the pressing, squeezing, or traumatizing of the Dim Mak Points (Vital Points); organ-piercing blows; blood gate attacks; traumatizing nerve plexus; and combinations thereof.

These fighting methods taught how to defend oneself by injuring, incapacitating, or even killing one's opponent. One of the highest levels was the complete understanding of Vital Point, Pressure Point or Dim Mak striking methods.

Some texts talk about 36 vital points, while others talk about 22 (16 on the front of the body and 6 on the back) vital points. The main thing you want to understand, is that many of the points you see on the different charts, will cause trauma to different degrees, no matter whether you believe in 36, 22 or any other number of points.

There are 3 separate categories of Dim Mak striking and they are:

a. **Tien Ching-** Attacking the Nerves
b. **Tien Hsueh-** Striking the Blood Vessels
c. **Tien Hsing Chi-** Attacking the Chi Meridians

Level One: Tien Ching, This method is where you attack the nerves of the body in order to induce paralysis.

This method works extremely well without even concentrating on any specific points, as you can find nerves all over the body and they can be struck, gauged, twisted, and poked quite easily.

As a matter of fact, just pick out a part of your body and start to dig into the area. Dig in at different angles and pressure levels. You will notice the pain factor rising depending on the amount of pressure you place on the area. Note: hitting or striking hard at a 45 degree angle on a nerve point you focused on, will result in actually causing damage to that person struck.

Some People Will Not Respond

One important thing to consider is some people don't respond to nerve strikes. There are a lot of reasons for this and some are but not limited to:

1. They are in excellent mental and physical condition and may have a very high pain threshold.
2. The locations and densities of their nerves are different than expected.
3. They are overweight and have a lot of fat covering the nerves, making them easier to miss.

Big Muscles, Big Target

An important point is that muscular people usually have their nerve points very close to the top of the skin since they have more muscle than fat built up. This should give you a good idea of how to beat someone, who is more muscular or perceived stronger than what you are. It is not always strength and muscle, but how precisely your strikes are placed on the opponents' body that determines the outcome of the fight.

Level Two: Tien Hsueh, This is the Blood vessel striking method, designed to seal the veins and arteries and cause blood clots.

When you strike an opponent in order to seal his blood vessels, death can be delayed through variations of pressure points and time sequences, which affect the blood flow. The majority of the time this particular method is used with internal chi striking. By sealing the blood, death will result because you do the following:

1. Block the circulation of blood to the opponent's major organs resulting in organ deterioration.
2. Cause blood clots which will travel through the body's circulatory system causing either cardiac arrest if the clot enters the heart or a major stroke if they enter the brain area.
3. Attack the main organ or gland when it is full of blood in order to immediately destroy it.

This can be achieved by knowing the precise time of day in which to strike the appropriate spot on the body in order to get the desired effect.

This is a very detailed and tricky method to learn, as it requires knowing time of day, location and using your internal chi energy in the correct manner. It is not in the scope of this course to go into complete detail with that particular method.

Level Three: Tien Hsing Chi, This is where you attack the Chi Meridians of the body in order to cause death immediately or within a specific time period.

Striking the electromagnetic flow of chi in the body is altered by "chi manipulating" the different bioelectrical fields of energy surrounding and permeating the body's structure. The purpose of this is to attack and destroy the four levels of energy that flow within the body. This requires the ability to externalize your chi (see **Chi Power Plus** and **Advanced Chi Video** for more info). This is one of the most dangerous practices and is considered one of the higher levels of striking you can achieve. You can only learn more about this specific method in our Inner Circle closed system part.

36 Deadliest Points on the Body

As mentioned before, there are several different thoughts on the deadliest points on the body to strike, but one thing is certain, all of the points shown in the diagrams and charts in this course are Dim Mak points.

 When hit with the right amount of force, angle and direction, these points can induce bleeding, fainting, increased blood pressure, the piercing of a major organ and or nerve plexus. This type of trauma can cause temporary numbing effects, paralysis or even death.

This information was formulated based on ancient acupressure points in the body. They would stimulate the points on either animals or humans. It is very well known, that tests of Dim Mak striking on different kinds of animals and even prisoners were used in the past, to test & prove the points to see if they indeed worked reliably.

The 36 points should be greeted with caution, as severe trauma will occur when you press, squeeze or strike one of the points in any hard or focused manner.

Most people think that Dim Mak striking is just that…striking. This couldn't be further from the truth. A lot of the most effective use of these techniques is when you can really dig or manipulate at different angles into the specific nerve point.

Sometimes these strikes can be used with a time delay effect to:

1. Block the blood circulation
2. Close the chi pathways to the bodies meridians
3. Attack the major nerve functions

When striking to the points using chi, results can be determined by the following:

1. A heavy focused strike can cause an immediate serious effect
2. A moderate strike will produce the effect within 3 days
3. A light strike will produce an effect in 30 days with the right mind intent

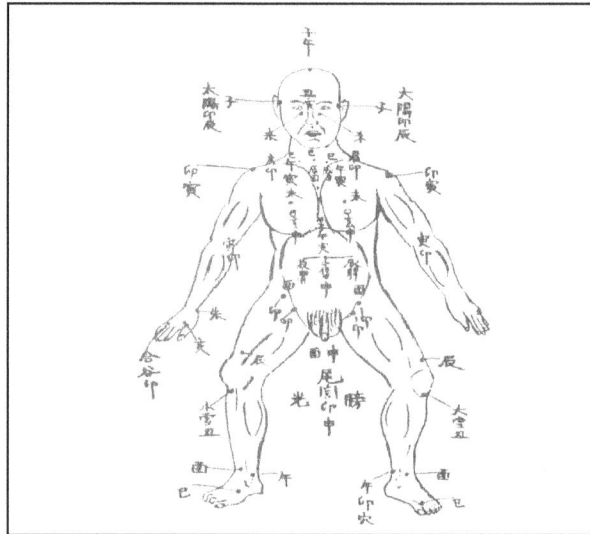

The picture above shows the original 36 deadly vital points. Notice the placement of the points. The points are both upper body and lower body with no back points.

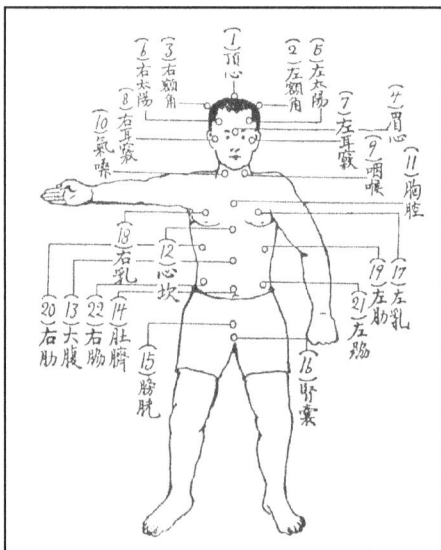

Another Chart of the 36 points (Front)

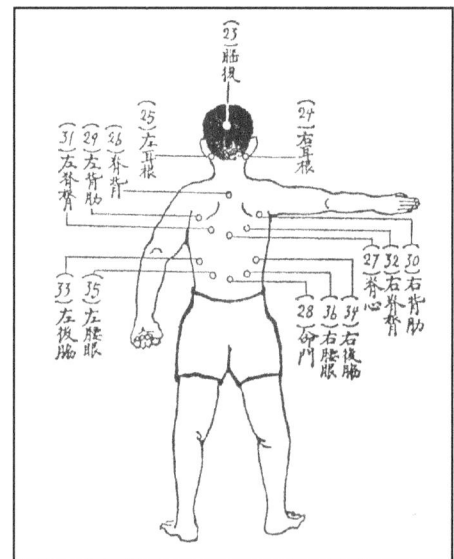

Same 36 Chart (Back)

As you can clearly see, the interpretation of which 36 points are the most dangerous or vital is up to the school of thought or even the instructor.

The next chart will show you the 36 most deadly striking points on the body depicted on our own "Redman" chart.

All of the 36, we have listed are vital striking points, but not all are Dim Mak points. The difference is that a vital point can be something as simple as the eyes or throat, whereas the Dim Mak points correspond to the actual gland or organ you are trying to penetrate.

Each point is described on the next page with our chart.

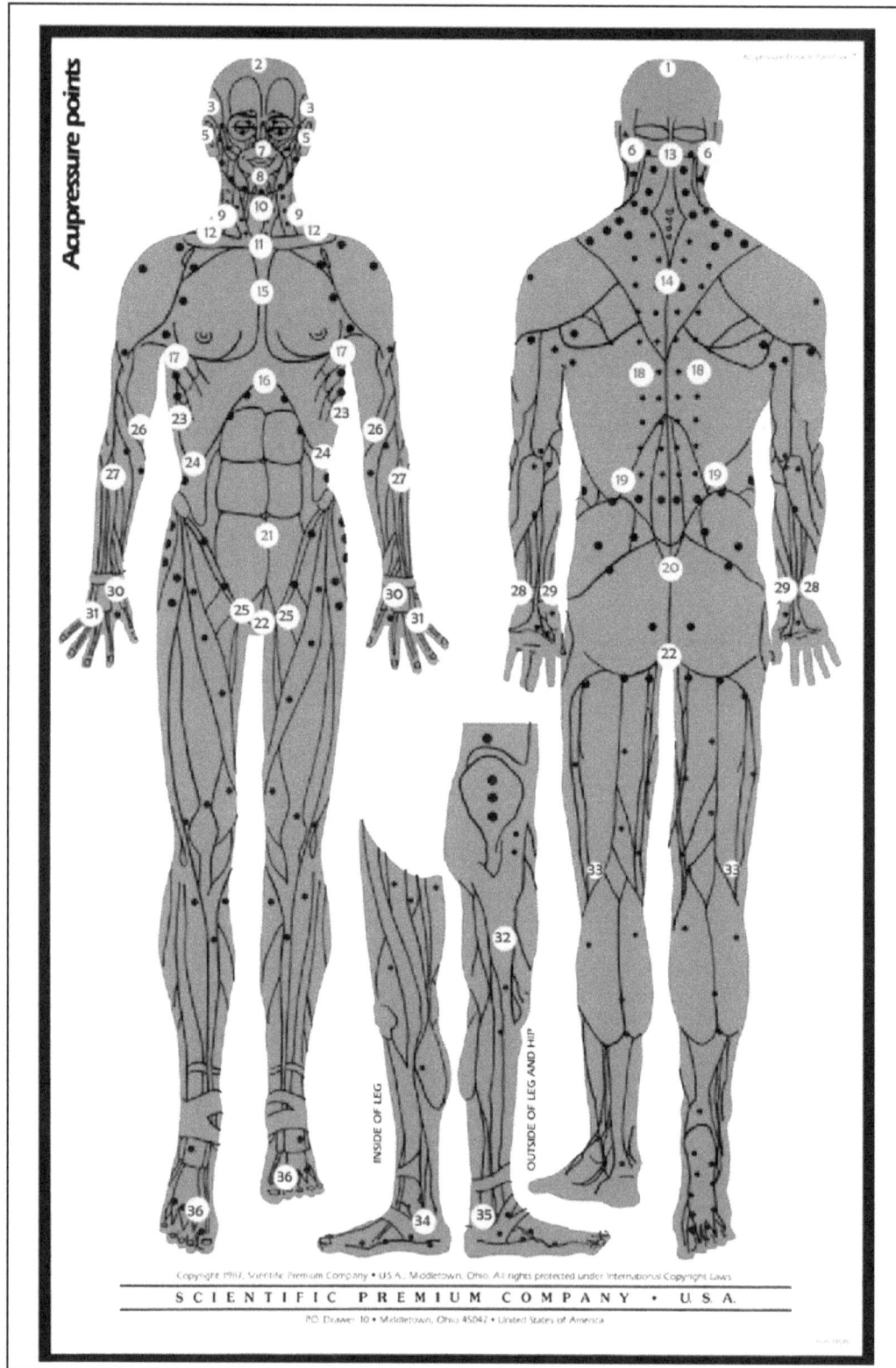

Acupressure points

INSIDE OF LEG

OUTSIDE OF LEG AND HIP

SCIENTIFIC   PREMIUM   COMPANY   •   U.S.A.

P.O. Drawer 10 • Middletown, Ohio 45042 • United States of America

The Thirty Six Vital Points

1. Coronal Suture
2. Frontal Fontanel
3. Temples
4. Eyes
5. Ears
6. Mastoid Process
7. Philtrum
8. Chin Indentation
9. Neck (Both Sides)
10. Throat
11. Sternum Area
12. Clavicles
13. Posterior Midline
14. Seventh Vertebra
15. Breast Bone
16. Xiphoid Process
17. Armpit
18. Fourth Thoracic Vertebra

The Thirty Six Vital Points

19. First Lumbar Vertebra
20. Tip of the Coccyx
21. Below the Umbilicus
22. Testicles
23. Seventh Intercostal Space
24. Tip of the Eleventh Rib
25. Inguinal Region
26. Biceps
27. Forearm
28. Wrist Crease
29. Wrist Crease
30. Hand (Between Thumb and Forefinger)
31. Hand (Web between the baby and ring finger)
32. Lower Thigh
33. Back of the Knees
34. Ankle (inside)
35. Ankle (outside)
36. Foot (Crease between the second and third toe joint)

In order to get proficient at these 36 points, you make them a part of your current martial arts curriculum. You should be able to work the points into the current striking technique set you currently do.

Practice is the key and that is what we are going to show you next.

Striking Methods

When the science of Dim Mak was first discovered, the original adapters, didn't use their hands to attack the points, but instead carried with them a device to strike to the Dim Mak points.

Keep in mind that you can use improvised weapons on these points such as ballpoint pens, sticks or martial art devices like the kubotan. There are many different types of striking methods and we are going to cover the most popular and how you will use them to strike at the points.

Once you realize the potentially lethal force that your hands can deliver to an opponent, you will come to appreciate the potency of this technology.

Penetration

Striking with the most penetrating part of the hand will be the most effective type of strike. Although most people use their entire fist in most fighting situations, we are going to show you how to use some very precise weapons to penetrate into the point.

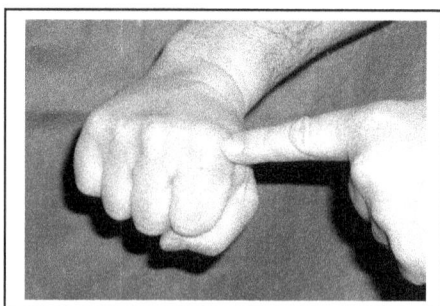

The Fist Strike

The most common strike to man is the fist strike. Ask anyone to make a fist and this is what they make.

For Dim Mak Vital Point Striking, you want to use the knuckles to penetrate into the point or nerves.

The amount of damage you do is based on the strength of the strike and the angle of penetration.

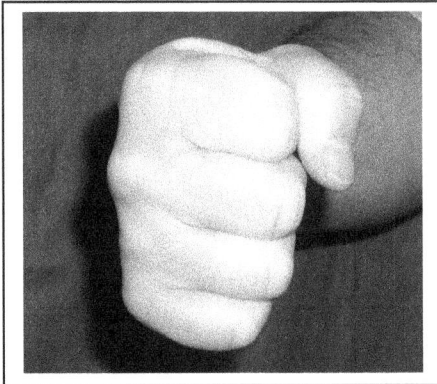

The Vertical Fist

Similar to the fist strike, but put in a vertical position. The emphasis is on the first two knuckles or the bottom two. This strike allows the flexing of the wrist to make the angle an upward or downward motion.

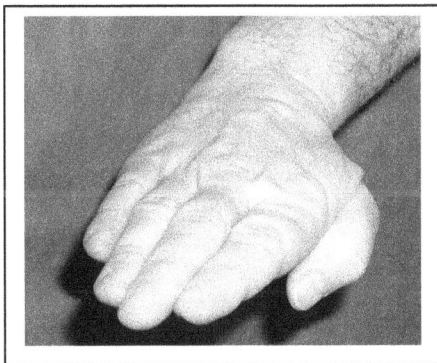

The Knife Hand or Thrusting Fingers

Thrusting the fingers into soft spots such as the eyes or lower stomach area work very well for Dim Mak Striking.

As you get better at hitting the points, you can use the fingertips as a tap on the point. Measure the blow to increase or decrease the damage.

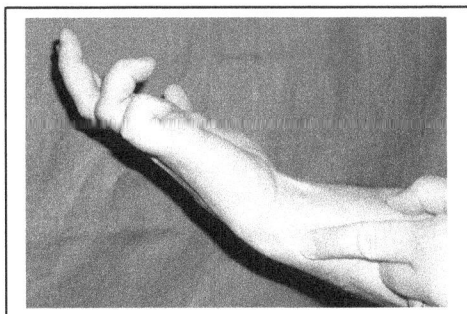

The Bone Chop

The picture points to the small bone on the wrist used for chopping actions. Works extremely well on the neck, arms, soft spots of the legs and back.

Using the entire blade of the hand somewhat dissipates the blow, so it is suggested to concentrate on striking with the small but powerful bone.

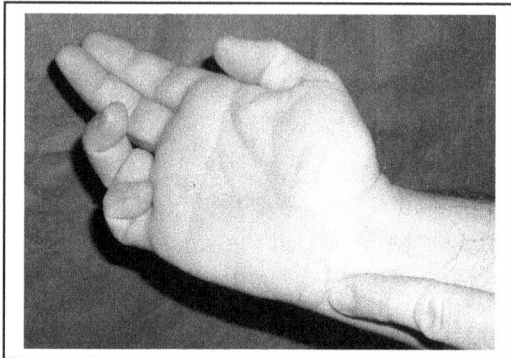

Palm Bone Strike

Similar to the Bone Chop, but this time you are using a palm strike utilizing the small bone pointed out in the photograph.

Used for downward or hooking striking motions. Works very well on the face and head areas. Make sure you are striking with the bony protrusion.

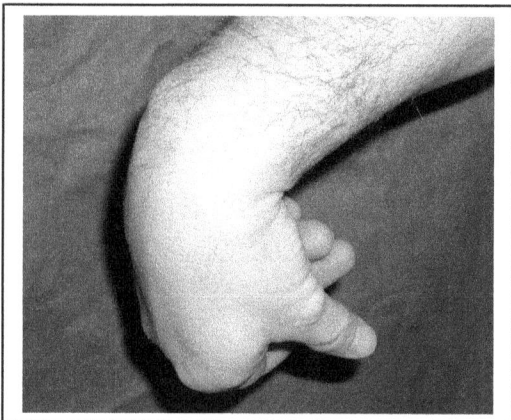

Crane Hand Strike

By using the bones on the wrist you can utilize the Crane hand strike. This is a very hard and penetrating bone that you can you can use to strike any soft areas of the body, especially the temples, throat, nose, arms and even parts of the legs.

This is used in a whipping fashion, so sometimes the motion is very much telegraphed.

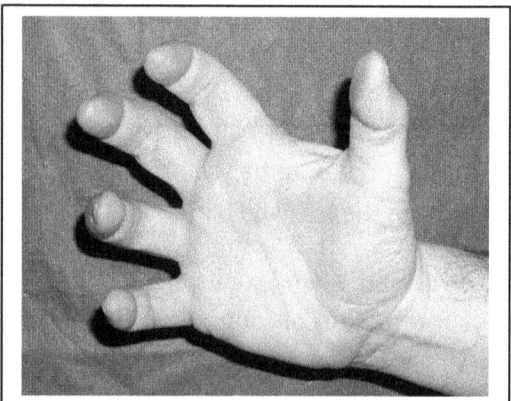

Claw Hand Strike

This strike can be used as more of an all-purpose strike hitting several points at the same time.

Used primarily for the face, using the fingertips to strike to soft areas.

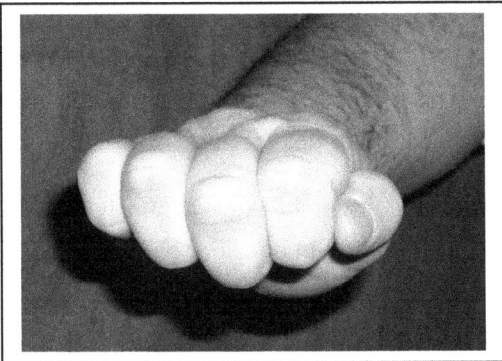

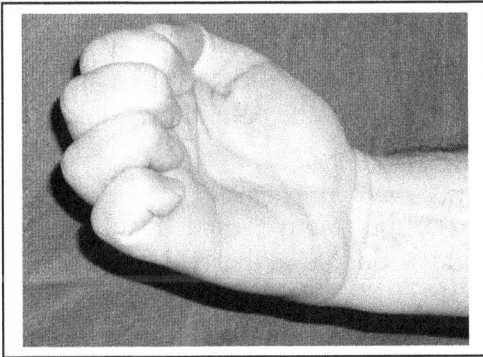

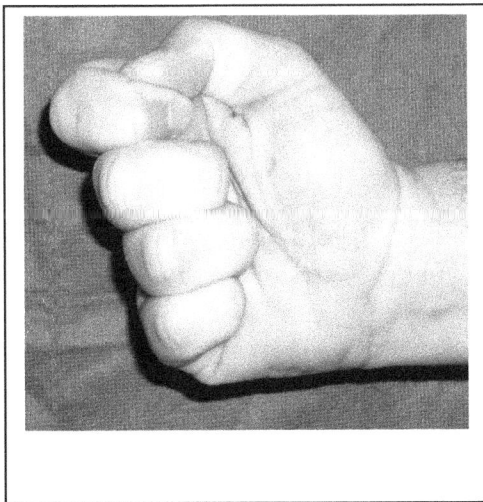

Leopard Paw Strike

The leopard paw is one of the most versatile strikes for Dim Mak. By using the fore knuckles of the hand in the configuration outlined in the pictures, you can penetrate a given area with one or all of the knuckles.

The leopard paw is also very effective as a chi strike that can travel to a specific organ or meridian point.

Knuckle Punch

This is one of the best strikes to use when doing Dim Mak striking. It can be used as an actual strike which is very effective in digging into a nerve point. It also allows you to rotate the finger into the point itself. This digging or rubbing action can be very effective when on the ground doing grappling maneuvers. It allows you to really get the angle on the right point, by moving the finger in a downward rotation.

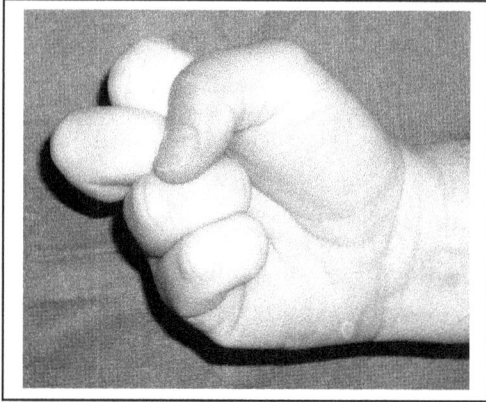

Middle Finger Fist

This can be used like the Knuckle punch and is a very penetrating strike, when thrown as a punch to soft areas such as the temple or neck.

It is a better back up than the knuckle punch in terms of the alignment, but does not have the angling ability like the knuckle punch.

Double Point Striking & Triple Point Striking

As you begin to learn these secret Dim Mak methods, you will want to learn the basics of the strikes and proper places to hit. Over time, you want to be able to hit one point or multiple points for increased abilities and results.

The information that follows is very much guarded information. Many would travel half way around the world (and some have) to learn these forbidden double and triple point striking methods.

By doing a double or triple point strike, you increase your ability to cause trauma to the opponent exponentially over just a single strike. The following chart has the location of the strikes and the description follows.

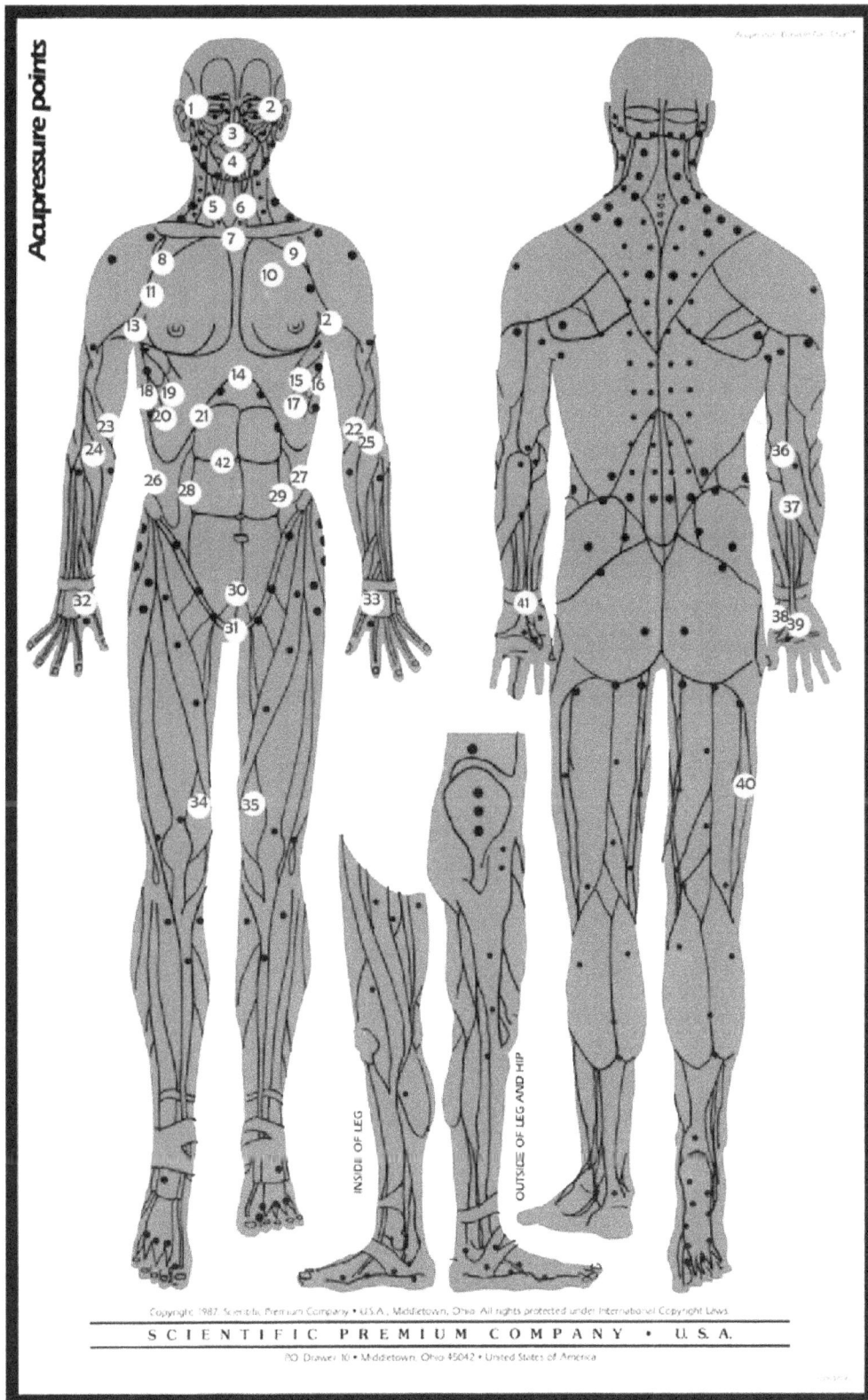

Acupressure points

INSIDE OF LEG

OUTSIDE OF LEG AND HIP

SCIENTIFIC PREMIUM COMPANY • U.S.A.

Guidelines for Striking

- If you strike one pressure point with the correct amount of energy and pressure, you will cause pain, and paralysis in that general vicinity; or a knock out depending on the area and point struck
- If you strike two of the points with the correct amount of energy and pressure in sequence, you will cause pain and trap energy inside the person's body, so the energy meets in the middle between both points, which will then affect the body's closest organ (to those points) adversely, as the access energy will then travel into that one organ or organs, depending on the points targeted.

Keep in mind that this is a general guide and that there are exceptions to the rule depending on the actual points you have chosen to attack. When you mix different combinations of Dim Mak points you will receive different body reactions. Here is a list of some double strike combinations.

1) #41 + #36: Paralysis of the Arm	1) #3 + #23 + #42: Death
2) #9 + #32: Paralysis & Cardiac Arrest	2) #10 + #4 + #27: Death
3) #10 + #4: Death by Cardiac Arrest	3) #41 + #37 + #4: Damage to heart and internal energy system. Possible death within 14 months.
4) #42 + #30: Knockout or Death	4) #41 + #23 + #6: Cardiac Arrest
5) #7 + #2: Knockout or Death	
6) #35 + #31: Knockout	
7) #41 + #6: Knockout	
8) #41 + #23: Knockout	
9) #6 + #17: Knockout	
10) #40 + #38: Knockout	
11) #6 + #20: Knockout	
12) #6 + #4: Knockout	
13) #6 + #28: Death	
14) #41 + #42: Knockout or Death	
15) #19 + #4: Knockout or Death	
16) #3 + #2: Knockout	
17) #22 + #12: Knockout or Death	

Training Methods

Most books and videos on the market pertaining to Dim Mak, Vital Point Striking, Pressure Points, etc, usually do an excellent job of describing the points and describing the effects you get from striking, but don't tell you how to train to be proficient with these kind of techniques.

We want you to learn some of the training methods that we have found to be very effective when used in the proper manner.

The first thing you need to do is put in the time to become good at this. You must study these charts and then practice using the striking methods from your particular martial arts. Many of the different martial arts out there have katas or forms. Many of these katas or forms were designed specifically to strike at vital points.

On the other hand, you can put your own unique sets of combinations together, in order to also get the desired results. The key is to keep an open mind while training and teach your mind to grasp the concepts.

Shadow Boxing

The ancient Shaolin Monks used a method of shadow boxing when they were doing their morning exercises. These exercises became the forms that later became what we know as the martial arts.

These shadowboxing sessions were designed for them to use their techniques against imaginary opponents. You can utilize this same concept with the Dim Mak striking techniques.

Some students have built training dummies with the marked vital points in order to practice their techniques. Others have placed round stickers from an office supply store on a heavy bag to simulate the correct point locations.

One way or the other, you must internalize the proper position of the points, so that you can increase your proficiency

Muscle Memory

You must burn this information into your brain. This is called building muscle memory. Muscle memory is where you train the body and the mind to react under certain guidelines that you control.

Becoming good at Dim Mak striking is reliant on getting your muscle memory down to the point that you will know where to strike, even under the most serious of circumstances. When trained properly, you will get your body to kick in the way your muscle memory was taught to it. This will allow you to respond with the appropriate strikes you trained your mind to deliver.

Diamond Point Striking Chart

One method that works extremely well is to put together a Diamond Point Striking Chart. You should design it like the one below. The points should be about the size of a pencil eraser head.

Once you have it set up, place it somewhere you go in and out of daily. Some put it on the side by their doorway to their room or office. The key is that every time you go in or out of the room you simply strike onto the points with your knuckles or other parts of the hand.

It doesn't have to be hard, just routine. Do it regularly and you will effectively teach yourself the ability to hit the pressure points you want to in an exact manner. Simply by doing this effective exercise, you can slowly teach your body & mind to be more precise. As a matter of fact, this is a secret method of training in order for you to burn into your muscle memory, the act of vital point striking.

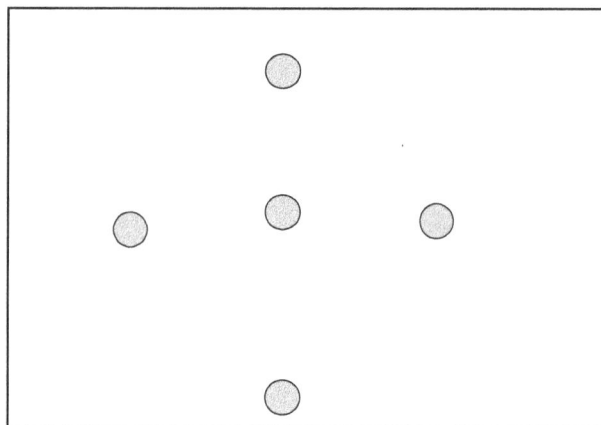

Sometimes it is the simplest training that will allow your skills to increase. This exercise is definitely one of those types.

Summary

Make sure you use caution when using these type techniques. You will find that when you use them in a healing way, that you will experience the joy of helping someone rather than hurting them. Like a double-edged sword, these concepts can hurt or heal. You are the one that must decide how to use them. These type techniques should be used to help your fellow man and used in a hurtful way, only as a last resort.

Part II:

Pressure Points

By Scientific Premium Company-USA

Published by Velocity Group Publishing

PO Box 9516 Hamilton, NJ 08650

> **"A wise man ought to realize that health is his most valuable possession and learn how to treat his illnesses by his own judgment. – Hippocrates, founder of modern medicine**

INSTRUCTIONS FOR THE SPC-USA ACUPRESSURE ERASABLE PAIN CHART

What is Acupressure?

Acupressure is firm, controlled and timed pressure applied by thumb, fingers, or elbow, on specific pain-causing "sore" spots of the muscles. No drugs or other medicines are used. "Sore" spots are actually a pattern of small knots, which constrict the flow of blood and oxygen, causing a painful muscle spasm.

Acupressure is both safe and healthful. Simple pressure on the constrictive knots will melt them, to free the flow of blood and oxygen. The acupressure therapy is momentarily painful. Pain should be controlled by a variance of pressure to individual tolerances.

On completion of acupressure and suggested muscle-stretching exercises, the very source of the pain is usually removed - often permanently – and blood circulation is enhanced in the areas treated.

Heavily muscled people will require more pressure than babies or the elderly. If the spot is extremely sore and tender, several mild applications of acupressure, over a period of time, can be used. Remember, you press each spot only as hard as can be reasonably tolerated.

For shoulder, back and seat areas, an elbow rather than thumb or fingers may be used. Also, when a smaller person, such as a child, is erasing spots on heavy-muscled adults, an elbow can generate the required pressure to erase pain. When pain is being erased from cramped muscles, the pain may move from one place to another - temporarily - even some distance away. Search for sore spots near the new pain location, and erase them. Don't get discouraged. Remember you are not merely masking pain, as with drugs. Instead, the pain erasure can be permanent!

Temporary pain relief is immediate, but easy-to-do muscle-stretching exercises, as directed, are required for permanent pain erasure. Stretching twice per day for several days is usually required.

Severe cases may require muscle-stretching exercises over a longer period of time. Following surgery of any type, acupressure should be used to speed the healing process, and relieve pain. It should be started even before stitches have been removed.

The major spots to be pressed are shown on the Chart as black dots. Sore spots may be found in other locations. The entire muscles in a painful area should be searched for constrictive knots or sore spots.

If pain is not erased by following directions on the SPC-USA Erasable Pain Chart, you should consult a physician.

Basic Directions

Press spots shown as black dots on the Poster to check if they are sore. Apply pressure to sore spots only; pressure on other spots is not necessary unless otherwise indicated. Note the shape of the muscle structure, and check the area around the shown dots to see if there are sore spots. Apply pressure, and hold it to sore spots only. Check the entire length of the muscle.

PRESS EACH SORE SPOT ON HEAD, HANDS, AND FEET FOR 5 SECONDS. COUNT OUT THE 5 SECONDS: "one-thousand-and-one, one-thousand-and-two, one-thousand-and-three, one-thousand-and-four, one-thousand-and-five".

PRESS EACH SORE SPOT ON NECK, SHOULDERS, TORSO, ARMS, AND LEGS FOR 7 SECONDS. COUNT OUT THE 7 SECONDS: "one-thousand-and-one, one-thousand-and-two, one-thousand-and-three, one-thousand-and-four, one-thousand-and-five, one-thousand-an d-six, one- thousand-seven".

JUST BEFORE GENTLY RELEASING THE PRESSURE, MOVE YOUR FINGER, THUMB, OR ELBOW IN A "+" SHAPE.

The average pressure is 5 pounds on head and neck; 10 pounds on hands and feet; 16 pounds on shoulders, torso, arms, and legs; 30 pounds on seat. You can check the amount of pressure you are using by pushing down on your bathroom scales. The amount of pressure applied should be adjusted to individual tolerances.

Warning! Pain medication (even over- the-counter) can erase the acupressure and corrective exercise therapy on your muscles. Drugs work to ARTIFICIALLY stimulate circulation and relax muscles. The MUSCLES can quickly become drug dependent because they are artificially relaxed. They can then revert to old, painfully constrictive memories and again cause muscle spasm.

DO NOT GIVE UP TOO SOON. Be sure you have followed the complete muscles when searching for tender spots. Sore spots, particularly in adjoining areas, or anywhere on the body, could be the trigger mechanism causing the pain. Include armpits and under groin in your search. The "rule of thumb" for number of acupressure treatments needed is one *for* each decade (ten years) of age. Be sure you have followed the exercises specified for each area, at least twice a day for 4 or 5 days.

If you are trying it on yourself, you may not be pressing hard enough to melt the constrictive knots. Ask a friend to help you. If a spot is extremely tender, apply heat with massage, heating pad, or a warm shower, before using acupressure, Acupressure applied with Chi-generated heat works best (see SPC-USA Chi Power Chart).

Stop Pain, Swelling and Bruising or Bumps and Sprains with Acupressure

As soon as possible after a bump, bruise or sprain begins start using the acupressure. DO NOT APPLY ICE! Ice constricts the blood flow and will actually retain swelling and bruising in the affected area. You must begin treatment immediately on injuries if you want fast results.

FIRST: Elevate the injured part high enough to allow the blood to flow back to the heart and lungs. The idea is to push the accumulated blood out of the injured area.

SECOND: Begin at the edges of the injury and apply pressure with your thumb. Hold each spot for the 5-7 seconds. The process is quite painful, but the results are worth it. Work your way around to the very center of the injury, even if the skin is broken (cover an open area with a sterile bandage first).

THIRD: You may have to apply hard pressure several times over a period of several minutes, depending upon the extent of injury. It is best if someone else applies the pressure, since the natural reflexes of the body may prevent you from hurting yourself that much.

FOURTH: Gently exercise the injured part while still elevated, and then while in normal position. After a short rest, you are free of pain and swelling, and back in action again!

These procedures can & should be followed even if a bone is cracked or broken. The Chinese set their bones in this manner. Each day they carefully examine the position of the bone to assure that it is growing back in exactly the right position. When the bone is put in a plaster cast, this examination is impossible. We are not recommending that you should set your own broken bones. We are simply stating that it has been done by many with good results. Plaster does not allow the blood vessel massage necessary to stop pain and itching. You may have to use a restrictive form that can be removed daily for massage and examination; otherwise the bone may break a blood vessel and cause internal bleeding. When healing in this manner, it takes much less than the typical 6-8 weeks done in the normal fashion with a cast & medications.

Erasing a Tension Headache

Examine the drawing of the back of the head on the Poster. Note the line of dots which form a pattern at the base of the skull. Press each spot, and if it is sore, hold the pressure for 5 seconds, counting out the seconds.

Spread your fingertips about an inch apart, and beginning at the top of the head, press in a broad row to each ear. Again, beginning at the top of the head, press in a broad row down the back of the head, checking for sore spots, and holding each one for 6 seconds. Exercise: Upon completion, firmly massage the entire scalp with fingertips or butts of palms.

Now look at the drawing of the front of the head on the Poster. Start with the spot at the bridge of the nose between the eyes. If sore, press for 6 seconds, using finger or thumb. Then start at the dot shown above the left eye, and press upward toward the eyebrow. Now feel the bone structure around the eye cavity. Press all the muscles around each eye cavity firmly, holding for 5 seconds each.

The Exercise: Stretch eye muscles by opening eyes as wide as you can and closing them as tight as you can, 4 times. With eyelids closed, look up, look down, look left & then look right. Repeat 3 times.

Next, using your thumb and fingers, pinch across each eyebrow the entire width, holding each pinch for 5 seconds.

Again, using all your fingertips slightly spread apart, press in a row across entire forehead, checking for sore spots. Hold each one for 5 seconds. Exercise by: massaging forehead.

Using thumb and curved fingers, above and below jawbone, press along entire jawbone, from each ear to middle of chin. Press muscles around entire mouth, and hold each spot for 5 seconds. Exercise by: opening mouth wide and closing mouth tightly, 5 times.

Bend chin down and to the left, so that the muscles on the left side of your neck are easier to feel. With fingers and thumb, squeeze neck muscle from your left ear down to where it attaches to the left side of your collarbone at two points. Hold each squeeze for 7 seconds. Then place fingertips at top edge of collarbone and gently press skin and small muscles over the edge, reaching toward the underside of the collarbone. Start at the "v" of the collarbone, and move across to your left arm joint. Hold each tender spot for 7 seconds. You may find a real "oucher" that's been bringing your headache back again and again. Repeat the entire procedure for the right side of the neck.

Again, examine the muscle structure shown on the back of the neck on the Poster. Start at the skull and follow each of the muscles down to where they attach to your shoulder bones. Also check each spot across to your arm joints, pressing skin and small muscles over the edge, reaching toward the underside of the shoulder bones. Exercise by: moving head backwards, with chin in air; then forward, with chin down, to stretch neck muscles. Then rhythmically turning head to far left, then far right, gently increasing side vision. If movement is jerky, search for additional sore spots. Forcefully shrug your shoulders several times.

If your job requires your being in one position for long periods of time, such as watching a computer screen, try to 'develop a habit of forcefully shrugging your shoulders several times during a work session. This will help prevent tension headaches from occurring.

Remove a Sinus Headache and Congestion

See front of head drawing on the Poster. Use the following steps to "drain sinuses" even if spots are not sore. Press the spot between the eyes, on the bridge of the nose, then upward against each eyebrow, and downward over tearducts. Search for sore spots around each eye cavity. Then press spots ON FACE down each side of nose. Hold each spot for 5 seconds. Press inward toward nose flange and hold 5 seconds. Exercise your eyes by opening wide and shutting tight, 4 times. Then with eyelids closed, look up, look down, look right, look left, 4 times.

Now with your finger or thumb, feel the skull bone across the middle of each cheek toward each ear. Press up and under edge of cheekbones, holding 5 seconds each. Massage cheeks. Search for sinus cavities above each eyebrow. Hold each spot for 5 seconds, then massage the areas. Next, using fingertips, slightly spread apart, press in a line from each eye to each ear.

Next, start with the spot at the jawbone hinge, and press in a circle around each ear, pressing firmly against the skull, and holding each spot for 6 seconds. Exercise by opening mouth wide, then closing mouth tightly) 4 times.

Now lean your head horizontally to the left and hold it there for 15 seconds. Then lean your head horizontally to the right and hold it there for 15 seconds. This is to drain your inner ear passages.

You should now be free of a sinus headache, with your sinuses clear and breathing easy.

Remove a "Migraine" Headache

Use fingertips slightly spread and press across entire top of head. Hold each spot 5 seconds. Now using fingertips, press all muscles above each ear. Hold 5 seconds. Do both sides of head, even if pain is only on one side. Massage top and sides of head firmly. It is important to press firmly enough to melt the constrictive spots, to free the flow of blood and oxygen. You should now be free of the "migraine" headache. If not, follow instructions and Exercises for Tension Headache.

Eye Ache

(1) Pinch eyebrow between finger and thumb, the full length of each eyebrow.

(2) Press upward next to nose cavity against eyebrow.

(3) Press spots around each eye. Hold each tender spot 6 seconds.

Exercise: Close eyelids, and look up, down, right, and left, 3 times. If pain persists, do spots for Tension Headache.

Earache

(1) If pain is in right ear, lie down on left side with left ear against pillow, for at least 15 seconds, to allow right inner ear to drain. (If in left ear, do opposite.)

(2) Press in a line around each ear, on the muscles which attach the ear to the skull.

(3) Pinch any sore spots on ear between thumb and finger (every place where you can pinch the ear) for 5 seconds each.

(4) Earache may be caused by wax buildup. You can get wax remover at a pharmacy. If ear is itching inside, see a physician for skin allergy medicine. Often a couple of drops of warmed extra virgin olive oil will help.

Mouth

Prior to and after a visit to your dentist, press around your mouth area, both inside and out. Acupressure the corners of your mouth, then stretch your mouth muscles by opening the mouth wide (you should be able to get your fist inside your lips) and closing tightly, repeat the process several times. Also, you should acupressure the inside of your mouth (gums and cheeks) after any dental procedure.

The mouth muscles can have harmful effects over your entire body. Replace missing teeth before you develop unhealthy symptoms because of jaw displacement. Any type of jaw injury is a potential for health problems.

Shoulder Pain

Shoulder pain is perhaps the most difficult pain to remove. It requires someone to apply the acupressure for you. These are the instructions for the applier.

Begin by checking the spots as you see them on the back of the body drawing on the Poster, and on the front of the body drawing, in the shoulder and neck area. Take your thumb and forefinger and press firmly each spot along the entire neck muscles between head and shoulder-front, side and back. Press over the edge of the top of the shoulder blade all the way to the arm joint.

Next, lift the subject's arm, and beginning at elbow, pinch back of arm muscle all the way to armpit. Pinch firmly, holding sore spots for 7 seconds each. Then using your thumb, or fingers, search the entire armpit for sore spots. Press each sore spot firmly for 7 seconds. Do both arms and both armpits even if only one shoulder is in pain. Also pinch along the entire muscles at the front and back of the armpits-upper arm to chest, and upper arm to back. Pinch firmly, holding each sore spot for 7 seconds.

Now press along sides of subject's body – the spots along the ribs - holding each sore spot for 7 seconds. With thumb and finger, pinch along entire front side of arm muscle, between shoulder and elbow, pinching each sore spot firmly for 7 seconds. Do other arm.

Now have the subject lie on the floor or table, face down, and check along both sides of spine, from shoulders all the way down (see the two rows of dots on the Poster).

Check for sore spots at the lower edges of the shoulder blades. Firmly press the skin against the edge and under the shoulder blade. Hold each sore spot for 7 seconds. If you have trouble locating the lower shoulder blade, have the subject move arm slightly up and down, or twist slightly, so that shoulder blade is seen.

Now have the subject sit up. Check for sore spot in middle of shoulder blade (not shown on Poster). Stand at side of subject, facing opposite direction. Put one wrist under subject's arm and lift upwards, while using other elbow to press on spot in middle of subject's shoulder blade. Hold 7 seconds. Now move to other side of subject and do other shoulder blade.

Exercise One: Now have subject stand up, and stretch left arm straight out to left, palm up and open, with thumb pointing as far backward as possible. Very slowly rotate hand as far as possible while breathing out. Very slowly breathe in while rotating hand back to the starting point. Do this 4 times. Do the same with right arm, 4 times.

Exercise Two: While standing, subject should clasp hands behind neck, and stretch elbows as far backward as possible, then move elbows as far forward as possible. Repeat 3 times.

Exercise Three: Subject must shrug shoulders at least 4 times, several times during the day. Really shrug them. With head and neck stretched as high as possible, pull shoulders as low as possible. Then, push shoulders as high as possible, while lowering head as far as possible.

The subject should be free of shoulder pain if you have searched the entire muscle areas, and erased all sore spots, and the subject has followed the exercises.

Chest Muscle Pain

(Lessens Severity of Chronic Angina and helps breathing)

(1) Keep head and chest elevated. If breathing is difficult, use bent forefingers to press at both sides of bottom of ribcage, pressing slightly up and under the bottom ribs. Hold for 7 seconds. (2) If you can generate Chi Power, gently hold the palm of your hand over the sufferer's chest where pain is most severe, and direct Chi there. Have the subject purse lips to inhale slowly, then exhale slowly. (3) If subject has had heart surgery, you will need to check all muscles between the ribs for sore spots. Especially, in the center, front and at the sides. Using thumbs or fingertips, press entire ribcage across chest from center front, around side, to spine in back.

Exercise: Hold fists together on front of chest. Then swing elbows back as far as possible. Straighten arms fully outward to sides, hands open while slowly inhaling. Return to starting point, while slowly exhaling. Do four times. NOTE: SPC-USA Chi Power exercises can greatly enhance circulation that will help build lungs and lessen angina symptoms.

Neck Muscle Problems

The neck muscle which starts just behind the ear lobe and attaches to the collarbone can be the cause of a lot of problems, including chest pain, ear aches, toothaches, or shoulder pain, even if you have no pain in the neck. It may have been caused by whiplash or by holding the head in the same position for long periods of time, such as watching a computer screen. It is also a difficult muscle to find on most people. To find the one on the right side, you must turn your face downward and far to the left.

Use bent forefinger and thumb to squeeze the muscle, or push against it with fingertips, to check for sore spots. Follow the muscle all the way to the collarbone where it attaches in two spots. Hold each sore spot for 7 seconds. Do both sides of neck.

Exercise: Sit on a chair and reach your right hand back to grab the middle of the back of the chair while you look as far to the left as possible. Then 10 bend head forward until chin touches chest, and stretch head backward as far as possible. Then reach your left hand back to grab the middle of the back of the chair while you look as far to the right as possible. Repeat each movement 3 times.

Upper Backache

See back of full body drawing on Poster. Check spots shown on shoulders and at base of neck. Check for sore spots at edge of and under shoulder blades. Check spots shown in two rows down each side of spine.

Exercise: Clasp hands on back of head. Move elbows as far forward as you are able, while slowly exhaling. Then move elbows as far backwards as you are able, while slowly inhaling. Repeat 4 times. Next twist upper body, hands still clasped to back of head, as far to left, then as far to right, as you are able, 5 times.

If pain persists, complete the following steps, and repeat exercises. Check neck for sore spots. Check armpits and sides for sore spots. Check entire head for sore spots. Complete steps for Lower Backache.

Lower Backache and Sciatic Pain

See back of body drawing on Poster. Check the spots shown as black dots where hip pockets would be in the seat area and spots on the buttocks. Check 8 spots on belt line (4 on each side of spine), and 2 above belt line. Check 3 spots down side of each hip (see drawing of outside of leg and hip). Pressing these sore spots requires using your elbow.

Begin at shoulders and press in two rows down each side of spine (as shown on Poster).

Exercise One: Lie on your left side and draw your right knee toward your chest, 5 times; lie on your right side and do the same with your left knee. Lie on your back and do same, 6 times for each knee. Also move your head forward to touch your knee. It is not necessary to actually touch head and knee "the purpose is to stretch the back muscles. Still on your back, arch your back and tighten seat muscles; hold for 10 seconds. Next tighten abdominal muscles; hold for 10 seconds.

Exercise Two; On hands and knees, arch your back like a cat as much as possible; hold 5 seconds; then wiggle shoulders and buttocks, to gently stretch back muscles. Then let your back (and abdomen) sag like a swayback horse as much as possible; hold 5 seconds; then wiggle again. Repeat 3 times.

Exercise Three: Still on your knees and left hand, move your right hand between your body and left arm and try to touch as far up on the left side of your back as possible. Repeat, balancing on your knees and right hand, and reaching with your left hand far up on right side of back. Repeat several times with each hand.

Menstrual Cramps, Pain in the Groin

See front of body drawing on Poster. Check spots shown in groin area and on fronts and sides of hips. Press against and under lower edge of ribcage, from center to sides, about one inch apart. Hold each sore spot for 7 seconds.

Then gently press on, over, and under edge of pubis bone (center of groin area) to search out and erase sore spots, by holding pressure for 7 seconds. Check for sore spots between legs under groin. (A pratfall could have caused the problem.) Then check for sore spots around navel (belly-button) and other abdominal muscles. Press spot above hip, moving skm and muscle down and inward over edge of hip bone.

Exercise One: Sit on floor. Put soles of feet together, 8 to 10 inches in front of body. Gently push left knee toward floor and then release it, 6 times. Do same with right knee, 5 times.

Exercise Two: Frequently throughout day, tighten anus orifice as if you were to draw water into the intestines. Push abdominal muscles outward while taking a slow, deep breath (as from two inches below navel); then tighten abdominal muscles while exhaling slowly. Next, place feet together and do several HALF KNEE BENDS with feet flat on floor.

If pain persists, follow directions for Lower Backache.

Cramps or Pain in Arms

Press all spots shown on arms. If pain persists, check the full length of each muscle for sore spots.

Exercise: Turn hands up and down, rotating wrists, 5 times. Bend and straighten arms, 5 times.

WARNING: This can also be a symptom for heart problems. If there is a doubt, check with a Medical Doctor. There are a number of very good medicines on the market to relieve heart-caused pain.

Elbow Pain (Tennis Elbow)

(1) Lay arm on table with palm down. (See front of body drawing on Poster) press middle spot at elbow and move in a line down to wrist, checking for sore spots. Erase them by holding pressure for 7 seconds.

(2) Press outer spot (see drawing) and move in a line from elbow to wrist, erasing sore spots.

(3) Press spot at elbow on inside of arm, and move in a line to wrist, erasing sore spots.

(4) Check the spot above elbow on inside of arm (see drawing), and move along curve of muscle to spot on outside of arm at shoulder cape, erasing sore spots. From this same spot, follow edge of shoulder cape muscle (shown on drawing) up to collarbone. Return from collarbone, across outside of shoulder to the same spot.

(5) (See back of body drawing) squeeze between thumb and fingers the full muscle of the back of arm, from elbow to shoulder.

(6) Check for and erase sore spots in armpit.

(7) Squeeze chest muscle at armpit.

(8) Squeeze back muscle at armpit. Exercise: Follow Exercises listed for Shoulder Pain.

(9) Check area around "funny bone" at back of elbow, and erase sore spots. (10) Again using your thumb and fingers, squeeze lower arm muscle, from "funny bone" down back/body side to wrist, then down back/outside of lower arm muscle. (II) Follow complete instructions and Exercise for erasing pain in hands.

Pain, Tingling or Numbness in Wrists or Fingers (often called "Carpal Tunnel Syndrome")

Follow instructions for Elbow Pain.

Stiff or Painful Arthritic Hands and Fingers

(1) Press all spots shown on palms and backs of hands.

(2) Squeeze sides, then top and bottom, along full length of each finger and thumb.

Exercise: Repeatedly bend and stretch fingers, gently bending all at once. Work up to completely bending and straightening each, one at a time.

Cramps or Pain in Legs

(1) Press each spot shown on legs.

(2) If pain persists, search the length of each muscle for sore spots.

Exercise: Holding onto a chair or table, bend both knees slightly and then straighten up, 5 times. Try to bend knees a little farther each time. Later, when legs and knees are more limber, you can stretch leg muscles by grasping one ankle while stretching other leg as far behind you as possible. Do both legs.

Knee Pain

(1) (See front of body drawing on Poster) check for sore spots in a straight line, from spot shown in middle above knee, to top of leg. Erase by holding 7 seconds.

(2) Check in line from inside spot above knee to groin.

(3) (See the outside of leg and hip drawing) check in line from spot above knee) to top of hip.

(4) Check entire area around and on top of kneecap for sore spots.

(5) This pain usually requires the help of another person. The helper should sit by your side and lift your leg over his. Then using an elbow, he may acupressure all points mentioned. He then must move on the other side of you, still in the sitting position, and repeat the procedure with his elbow on the outside of your leg. The elbow is broader and can be used with greater pressure.

(6) Have the subject lie on his stomach, and use your elbow on the muscles behind the knee.

(7) In most cases, you will need to do both knees and legs, even though the pain is only in one knee.

(8) Sometimes the pain is caused by toes, feet, ankles, shins, or calves. Be sure to check all of these areas as well.

Exercise: Place feet together and do several half knee bends with feet flat on floor. If your pain is too severe to do knee bends, lie on your stomach and have your helper grasp your foot and bend your leg back, gently increasing the length of the bend, each time. Do both legs, but one at a time.

Stiff or Painful Arthritic Feet and Toes

(1) Press each spot shown on feet and ankles.

(2) Squeeze sides, then top and bottom, along full length of each toe.

Exercise: Repeatedly bend feet up and down, then side to side, moving only at ankles, not at knees. Repeatedly stretch arches and toes. Remember to exercise in slow rhythmic movements. If movements are still jerky, search for additional sore spots. Have helper stretch the foot muscles by bending foot and then toes up and down and side to side.

Pain, Tingling or Numbness in Ankles or Toes (often called "Carpal Tunnel Syndrome")

(1) Begin at back of calf muscle, at spot shown in middle (see back of body drawing on Poster) and search for sore spots on entire back of leg, up to knee and down to ankle. Erase sore spots by holding pressure for 7 seconds.

(2) Search for SOTC spots from front of knee to ankle, on top and both sides of shinbone.

(3) Check around kneecap for sore spots.

(4) Follow instructions and Exercises for Feet and Toes. Note: Use hand to gently pull toes upward toward shin and then stretch toes back toward calf.

Relief of Pain from Hemorrhoids

Press spot at very bottom of tailbone, and hold 7 seconds. Press the skin to under the tip of the bone. You will know it is the right spot if it is sore. This does not remove the hemorrhoids, but it can stop pain, itching, or bleeding. They are usually a symptom of prolonged tension or anxiety, which has also affected your internal organs. The diligent practice of SPC-USA Chi Power can prevent recurrence.

Relief for Unwanted Habits, Anxiety, Stress, Tension or Anger

If used immediately, Steps (1) and (2) may do it. If not, use as many Steps as required.

(1) Take a slow, deep breath (see Deep Breathing Exercise).

(2) Open mouth, place thumb on inside of middle of left cheek, with forefinger on outside of same spot, and pinch gently but firmly. Hold 5 seconds. Do same on right cheek.

(3) Press spots on jaws, directly under ear lobes. If tender, hold for 5 seconds.

(4) Using thumb and forefinger of right hand, pinch left hand at point between thumb and forefinger, for 5 seconds. Reverse positions and repeat.

(5) Search entire head and neck for sore spots, pressing each one for 5 seconds. Then massage scalp.

Deep Breathing Exercise

Breathe very slowly, taking deep breaths, from below navel. Goal is to take 30 seconds to inhale and 30 seconds to exhale. Repeat 5 times. With practice, you can do it!

Yin/Yang Exercises

Move in a slow Yin Yang rhythm, to gradually increase your stretch. Yin (negative) releases, while Yang (positive) pulls. This can be done in time with slow music. If the movement is jerky, you still have problems. Search for additional sore spots and repeat stretching exercises with resistance, to build strength. Relaxed muscles should be mushy, but capable of becoming like stone on command.

Pressure Points for Protection

A sharp strike on any of the Acupressure Points can cause great pain. All of the Kata Forms are intended to strike another body at given angles over the pressure points shown on the SPC-USA Acupressure Chart. Sharp, hard pressure applied to two points, one very quickly following the other, magnifies the pain and can render a person unconscious. When you add Chi to the strike, the strike can go deeply into the body to affect his entire nervous system. A sharp finger strike on the center dot of the three large dots on the chest near the shoulder, can immobilize while still being conscious if rendered with quivering Chi. It can take the "fight" out of your enemy quickly.

There is a discipline called Tuite (tuweetay) that teaches exactly the correct angles to apply this hard pressure. Few teach the Tuite disciplines. They are very dangerous for the novice to use. All Tuite practitioners should be very well self-disciplined to not use this technique un-necessarily. Tuite requires strong study of inner muscle structure and nerve paths. Only the most devoted practitioner will learn this because it requires deep study of medical charts. Tuite is to be used only as a last resort to prevent permanent injuries.

Hard Contact Sports

Sharp blows or prolonged pressure applied on many of the points shown (LARGE DOTS, in particular) can cause muscle spasm, pain and immobility. The points to disable are (usually) over a knotted muscle. Anyone who has knotted muscles is subject to disablement in this manner. Therefore, a complete check of all points shown on the Acupressure Chart, is advisable prior to full contact sports. Whether due to hard contact sports, inactivity, or drugs, anyone can develop points that are repeatedly sensitive and will require repeated acupressure. Also, prior to competition, use the relaxation techniques to help you maintain better mental control.

Chinese Splits and American Splits

Before you begin this type of stretching exercise, you must first heat up your body till it sweats. Then start by stretching your neck muscles every time. Roll your head, to reach each neck muscle. You will not be able to achieve great success without stretching your neck first.

It's also a good idea to stretch your calf muscles before trying to work on the Splits. Stand with your back to a wall, and gradually inch your heels upward until you are standing on your tippy toes. Slowly inch back down. Repeat several times.

You must acupressure your leg and groin muscles every day. Try sitting down, with both legs stretched out to the sides, while you work the acupressure points in and around the groin area. Be sure you try to relax your muscles, trying not to tense up, while you apply the acupressure. Next, bend forward to try to touch your chin to the floor. Of course, it is only when you have become really stretched out, that you will actually be able to do this. Be sure that the first couple of times that you bend forward that you stay relaxed and arch your back. Keeping your back arched will help you stretch your muscles, but will help you avoid backache.

Only when you are fully relaxed will you feel serious pain while acupressuring the leg and groin muscles. Remember that after a few acupressure treatments and stretches, this pain will be significantly reduced.

Beginning stretchers should wait two days between hard stretches. Do only easy stretches on those two days. Acupressure every day!

More advanced students should stretch hard only on even days. Then on odd days, stretch easy and relax as much as possible while acupressuring leg and groin muscles. This is when the serious pain begins for most. Learning the Splits requires daily practice and daily acupressure!

Before you practice this leg stretching, acupressure the muscles in your leg and groin areas, to remove any knots you may have acquired. While you are practicing Splits, acupressure the groin or leg muscles that are in pain. You can then continue your stretch to an increasingly greater degree. After practicing, acupressure the sore muscles again.

Ballet dancers use a bar to stretch muscles. You can even use a wall to help learn this stretch. But, you should always use as much pressure with your thumbs on groin area spots as you can handle, to help with the pain of this very difficult exercise.

Common Household Remedies

All medicine is simply an aid to natural healing. The body heals itself. Medicine can often help. Acupressure and Chi Power are the best and least expensive of all healing methods. Olive Oil, preferably extra virgin olive oil, relieves chafing and itching from chapped skin, sunburn, and heat rash.

Distilled white vinegar gets rid of most fungus-caused problems (like athlete's foot). Baking Soda made into a paste, or added to your bath water, relieves allergies (such as mosquito bites) and sunburn. It is also an aid to healing cuts inside the mouth. Salt is also a major cleanser of wounds. Alcohol can help kill germs to prevent infection, but this also kills good bacteria. Plain water with very mild soap is the best cleanser over open wounds.

Live Plants

We inhale oxygen, and exhale carbon dioxide. Plants take in carbon dioxide and give out oxygen. For this reason, we need many live plants inside, especially in our work and sleep areas, as well as outdoors. Plants also absorb air pollutants.

Water

Drink plenty of pure water. You need the water to help your digestive and blood systems. Get a carbon filter and attach it to your drinking faucet, if necessary. Soft drinks, beer, tea, or coffee are not substitutes, and will require your drinking additional water to get rid of the residue they leave in your system.

Fat, Blood

Leviticus 3:17, "This is a permanent law throughout your land, that you shall eat neither fat nor blood", still applies to us today. In Old Testament days, God required that they be given to Him as a sacrifice. By taking it away from the people, God was protecting them from harm.

People who live in tropical, insect-infested areas develop a higher blood pressure and thinner blood, which increases Yang Chi, and protects them from insect bites. People who live in cooler climates have lower blood pressure and thicker blood, which increases Yin Chi, and enables them to easily draw animals, birds and fish to them.

Salt

Leviticus 2:13, "Every offering must be seasoned with salt, because the salt is a reminder of God's covenant." Many medical journals today warn against salt because they think it causes high blood pressure. But, salt and potassium are vital to your electrical system. A person that sweats too much salt from his body will die. Loss of potassium has the same effect.

Details for developing Yin and yang Chi Power are found in SPC-USA Chi Power Charts.

Part III

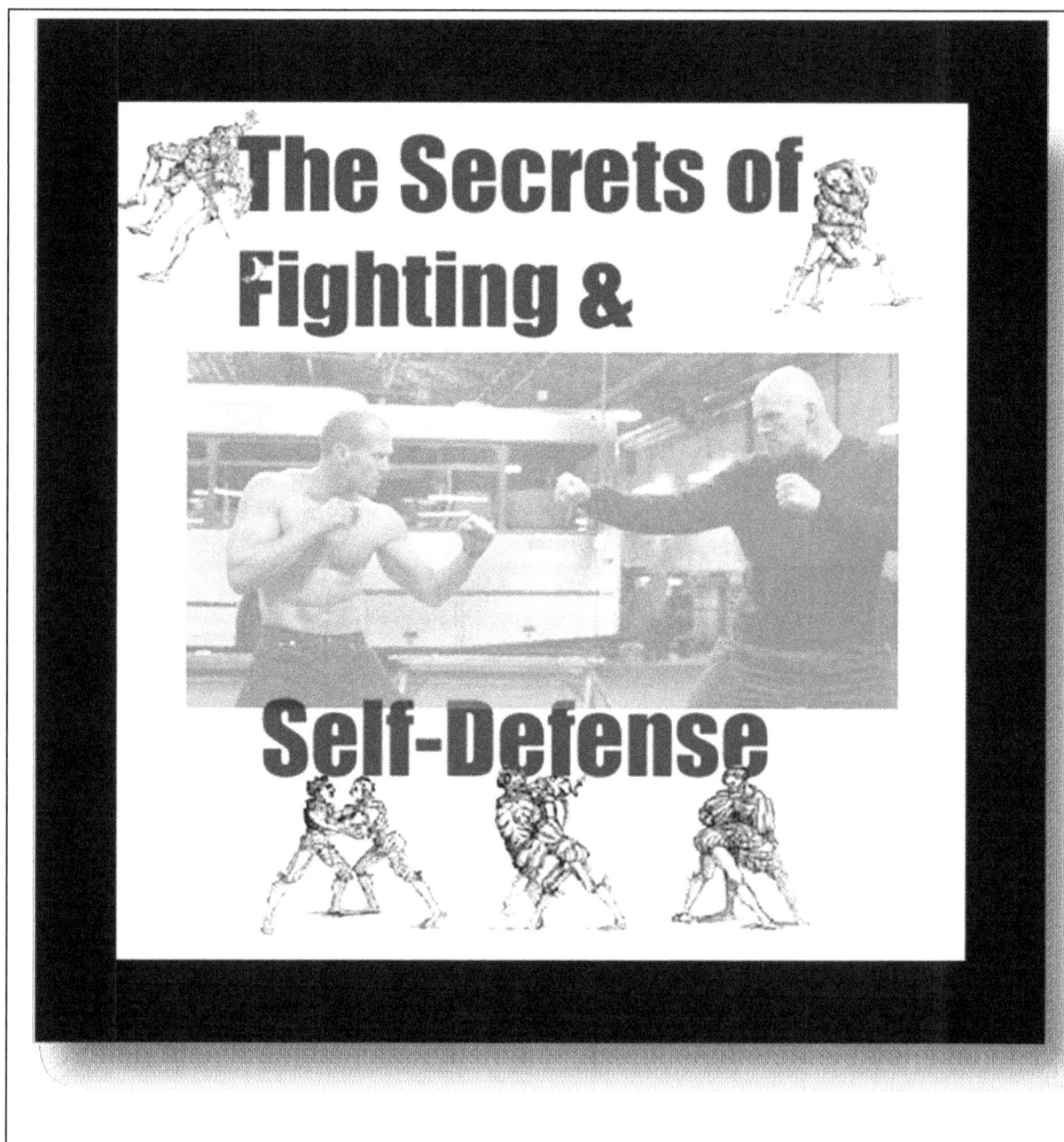

The Secrets of Fighting and Self Defense

The purpose of this manual is to instruct you on how to successfully defend yourself in a violent confrontation. This manual is not a substitute for a qualified instructor. You must take the concepts, methods and tactics described herein and apply them in practice, in order to get them to work in real life situations.

The techniques described in this manual can inflict bodily harm. We accept no liability for you using these techniques to hurt or intentionally or unintentionally end someone's life. These strategies are being offered for information purposes only.

FOUR ZONES OF ATTACK

Any true combative martial art must be able to meet all of the necessary ranges or zones of attack to be called a complete art. Unfortunately, most martial arts schools or methods only cover 2-3 zones at most! This leaves the art incomplete and leaves the practitioner at a dangerous disadvantage when it comes to the cold hard realities of street survival. Although the 4 zones of combat are important elements in the confrontation, the real key to being effective with a real life situation is the ability to harness the power of your mind and creating the mental toughness to come out of a confrontation in one piece.

The 4 zones combined with the mental training, gives you the tools necessary to defend yourself from all possible attack situations. We are going to look at all 4 zones and give you the reasons why you would bring the fight to each zone. Also, what the counters are in each zone as well. Every combat situation we are in is going to be different, being that circumstances and the location are hard to predict or dictate ahead of time.

We will also cover the different types of scenarios or fights that could happen in real life and what methods or tactics are used for each situation. A mugging is different from a bar fight, a fight with a friend at a party after too much drinking is also different from a multiple attacker confrontation. We will take and examine what must be done to effectively neutralize these different
situations and the most efficient manner possible, but first we will cover all 4 zones and how it is imperative to become proficient at each zone. The 4 zones are as follows:

1. **Boxing Zone**
2. **Kicking Zone**
3. **Grappling/Trapping Zone**
4. **Ground-fighting Zone**

Each zone has strengths and weaknesses, and no zone is the right zone at all times. They key to the 4 zones is being able to recognize and flow between zones when an altercation or confrontation changes, so you can adapt to what is happening to you. We will cover when each zone is the right zone to use and when it is the wrong zone to use.

BOXING ZONE

This is the first zone in fighting and the one that most people will go to, as this is our most natural thing to do in a fighting situation. Even children learn how to hit with their fists early on in life, so it would make sense that this is the first zone to become proficient in. They call boxing the "Sweet Science", because it is really knowing not only how to hit, but also knowing how not to get hit.

This is also the first zone because most confrontations take place in this zone, and many fights have been won or lost in this zone. A good boxer or street-fighter will hone their skills in this zone and will be able strike quickly and decisively with the needed power to end it fast.

This is why we have implemented the boxing drills and combinations into our arsenal of techniques, because on the street, boxing is the method of choice for most attackers. Boxing matches can be seen weekly and so it is easy for people to at least pick up some of the moves in this rudimentary manner.

Boxing skills are needed so that you can thwart through balance and sensitivity any boxer's ploys. It is also necessary you become aware of what those skills are, so that we can form a plan of action against an opponent that may have good boxing skills. One thing is for sure and that is:

"Most attackers will have poor boxing skills and will have a tendency to throw wide looping, hooks or round-house punches with little skill other than power".

In this first zone, blocking becomes imperative, in that if you can't stop the blows from raining in on you, you will never have a chance for a counter attack. This is where proper blocking and evading fundamentals are essential in order to defeat the sometimes stronger and more aggressive street attacker you might have to face.

Learn blocking not only in a defensive way, but you should be able to get offensive with the blocks, by the way in which you learn to block. The blocks should be at a 90 degree angle, and should be in a striking manner. You should tighten the arm right before impact to get the right desired numbing effect to the opponent's arms or legs. Always remember

"BLOCKS ARE STRIKES AND STRIKES ARE   BLOCKS"

The Box

The key to becoming a great fighter or martial artist is the ability to block and or avoid being hit. The Box is the necessary area to protect on the upper-body. The reason that this is being pointed out to you is that you must train yourself to keep your guard up, blocking the area within the box for protection at all times.

The box is an imaginary box that runs from the fore head to the bottom of the groin area. This is the area (make it a rectangle box mentally) you must protect from strikes or kicks.

Furthermore, it is not necessary to block outside of this box, which most karate styles teach you to do (with wide outward blocks), since strikes or kicks like that won't hit you in any vital areas.

Centerline Concept

Centerline is an imaginary line that runs down the center of your body. *Most of the vital targets on the body reside along the centerline such as, center eye brow, nose, teeth, chin points, throat, solar plexus, bladder, groin and others.* By using the box concept you are pretty much protecting centerline, but we feel that it is necessary to recognize where it is on you, as well as the significance of a target area like that, which is on an opponent.

This first zone is the range at which most confrontations are started in, and in a lot of cases where they end. Knowing the keys to protect the body in this zone is key and that comes back to what we would consider not being in **"target range"**, which means **never get closer than the distance at which your opponent can strike you with his hands.**

We have all seen a typical fight where two people face off at a close distance and start the traditional shoving match. This is absolutely the worst thing to do and is a good way to get **"Sucker Punched".**

The "Sucker Punch" is an excellent technique when you know that the action is going to start and you know that you want to come out on top. The ability to perceive the situation and knowing that it is time to move is every bit as important, as how to move itself. We have a saying that almost guarantees you winning about 90% of the fights you get into and is a simple tactic that works, because you are controlling the action from start to finish. This is one of the ways you can beat the stronger, faster, more seasoned opponent almost every time and the tactic is to:

"HIT FIRST, HIT FAST & KEEP HITTING"

This single concept will give you the knowledge that your action must be deliberate and to the point. No fuss no muss, just get in there, get the job done and get out of there. Some may say this is sneaky, but we are talking about a situation that we are looking to control, before it gets too far out of hand that you can't control it.

These techniques have to do with situations, where you have no other alternative, but to fight. This is after all your verbal methods have been used and you realize that it's either you or him. These methodologies work, and work well, but again these are techniques for self-defense not for picking street fights to see how tough you are.

If you really want to see how tough you are, remember that there is always someone better, tougher, stronger & faster than you. And of course every dog has their day, so keep that in mind if you're thinking of using these methods to fill your ego. Fighting for ego is the worst thing to fight for. As it is born out of a low self-image, and what you are trying to accomplish here is to increase your awareness and self image to create a boldness and confidence, not only for self-defense, but for everything that you do in life.

We will cover kicking zone next, but first we wanted to cover the fact that there are some low line kicks that work in the Boxing/ Zone that are instrumental to becoming a total fighter.

The kicks used most in this zone are the low line oblique kicks common to Wing Chun Kung Fu and Jeet Kune Do. These are destructive kicks done with the inside of the foot and would be best described as similar to how you would kick a soccer ball.

These devastating low shin or knee kicks work great in combination with your Boxing Skills. Learn to be able to attack the body or head (middle and high line), as well as the shin or knee (low line) at the same time, as it will give you an advantage over your opponent, since very few martial artists ever learn to do this well.

Below are some techniques to use in each zone to be effective. Here are some of the ways to defeat Boxing zone.

- ✓ **Pull back to kicking zone and use kicking techniques.**
- ✓ **Close the gap and enter into grappling/trapping zone.**
- ✓ **Close the gap and take person to Ground fighting zone.**

One of the things that you should try to avoid in fighting someone, is fighting them at their best zone or attribute. In other words, make sure that you are not trying to slug it out with someone that has a great amount of boxing skill, because if they are good at that zone, they will take you out before you even know what happened. We use a saying that I heard years ago and it still applies today.

"Never box with a boxer, never kick with a kicker, don't close the gap on a grappler, and never go to the ground with a ground-fighter."

Boxing Zone is the area that most people are aware of when looking at a physical confrontation, and should be drilled into you, so that you know your best attacks, as well as how to defend and react in a way that will make you successful in a confrontation.

KICKING ZONE

Kicking Zone is the area that most people associate with the martial arts, because of the many movies that show the Karate or Kung Fu man doing fantastic kicking techniques to the bad guys head to win their fight? This is not necessarily a realistic aspect to how real fights will be won.

Kicking Zone can be one of the best zones to carry out a successful self-defense situation, if you understand how to use it effectively to exploit your opponent's defense.

We can talk about a variety of kicks and kicking combination, but our emphasis will be what kicks are effective in a self-defense or "street" type of situation, not what looks pleasing or fancy. There are some arts that concentrate exclusively on high kicks to the head and upper body area, which is fine for sport and building up good flexibility and cardiovascular endurance, but really aren't designed for the realities of a violent confrontation.

We utilize kicks that can be taught to anyone at any age and don't require flexibility or years of practice and study to master. The ability to end the confrontation quickly and efficiently is our goal. That means using techniques that work well all of the time, not only in an ideal situation. We utilize "low line" kicking concepts that give the practitioner the most chance of winning on the street.

The low line is the area from the feet to the knee area, and in some cases the groin can be included in this as well. These are targets that are easy to get to and don't take an overwhelming amount of training to get good at (or flexibility). Our low line kicking will include but is not limited to strikes to the following areas.

- ✓ **Foot Stomps**
- ✓ **Kicks & Scrapes to the Shins**

✓ **Kicks to the Knees**
✓ **Kicks to the Thigh**
✓ **Kicks to the Groin Area**

Low line kicking enables even the smallest person a tactical advantage over a much larger attacker, since you are sticking to areas that most people will not be thinking of protecting. They can be struck with your kicks even before they realize what is happening!

Kicking Zone is a long-range weapon where you can reach your opponent with your feet, but they can't reach you with their hands. Again the concept of being able to move from zone to zone in order to be able to attack the opponent where they are the weakest or at least not prepared for is the key goal.

A good rule to go by while using low kicks, is you should always use the closest weapon to the closest target. In some schools, you can learn hundreds of kicks that look real flashy and can impress people, but what we are talking about is having a few good techniques (you pull from our little bag of tricks) that you can count on in a reliable way every time.

Why should you learn fancy high kicks when it takes years to learn them in the proper manner. Not to mention the fact, as you get older and older, it gets harder to do the same kicks that you did in your youth. As you age, your flexibility will decrease, meaning those high kicks become more and more impractical as you go along.

"The Best Way to Kick an Opponent in The Head Is When He Is On The Ground!"

You can learn the lower line kicks which take no flexibility or athletic ability, and virtually no maintenance. This is a secret of learning how to prepare yourself for combat no matter what your age is and/or whether you are in good shape or not.

Every zone is vulnerable and Kicking Zone is no different than any other zone, as it has its strengths and weaknesses. The strengths being that you will be able to execute quick decisive kicks to targets that are close enough to get to with your feet, but that your opponent will not be able to counter with his hands.

A good quick kick to the groin is one of the most effective strikes that you can deliver to stun an opponent and then finish them with other kicking and/or striking combinations. The downside to the Kicking Zone is that if the opponent is a savvy fighter, he can do several of the following tactics:

✓ **Angle off of the attempted kick and close the gap.**
✓ **Block the kick and counter with Boxing tactics.**

✓ **Close the Gap and enter into Grappling Zone.**
✓ **Avoid/block kick and take opponent to ground**

Again, the thing is you must remember is that a good kicker will get a kick off before you can realize what is going on. I have seen people do a kick to the groin so fast that is almost imperceptible to the human eye.

This is the type of technique that you want to get off on your opponent, but you don't want him to get off on you. That is why we emphasize the quick low line kicks that will give you that decisive edge in a combative situation.

Kicking, like any other skill you will develop will take a lot of time and practice in order to get good at hitting targets. Learn to get good at a couple of kicks that you can rely on in your time of need. The two kicks that you should get really proficient at are:

1. **Front snap kick to the groin**
2. **Oblique kick to the shin or knee**

Learn how to hit targets from different angles so that you will be able to call these skills your own.

No one has all of the secrets and nobody can really give you a certification of your own skills, that takes you working and honing these skills, so that you can call them your own. This is a "Master Key Concept" to the "Secrets of Self-Defense"!

TRAPPING/GRAPPLING ZONE

Trapping/Grappling Zone could probably be the most important zone to get proficient at, as it gives you a tactical advantage against most street-fighters, boxers, and in a lot of cases even martial artists.

This zone is not taught in a lot of schools and so the practitioner never realizes their full combat potential. More and more martial artists are realizing that you must have some type of infighting range to go to, so that you can end a confrontation quickly.

"Trapping/Grappling Zone is the ability to close the gap, and move from Kicking or Boxing Zone into a range that delivers a high intensity barrage of fists, elbows, knees, head-butts, arm locks, and chokes."

This zone is the one that you want to get to when you want to end the confrontation with finality. The key here is the ability to close the gap and put the opponent in a defensive posture, with a backward reeling motion that inhibits them from counter attacking. This gives you the forward motion needed to drive right through the opponent, causing them to lose balance and thus giving you the momentum to further inflict pain and damage.

To give more detail as to how Trapping relates to the martial arts, let's take a closer look at what exactly trapping is and what the advantages are in using them.

Trapping is removing or immobilizing obstructions in order to get a strike into a particular target area. Trapping is primarily used in **Wing Chun Kung Fu** and **Jeet Kune Do,** but is also used but referred to as sticking, checking or pinning within the **Chinese Kenpo** system.
Trapping is also used to trap the arms in a manner that will give you an advantage within a close range fight or confrontation.

There are many different types of traps that can be used within the Trapping/Grappling Zone, but we will just give you an idea of two that we will use the most within this system of fighting.

1. **Pak Sao- Slapping Hand**
2. **Lap Sao- Grabbing Hand**

To get to Trapping/Grappling Zone you must first go through either the Boxing Zone, Kicking Zone or both. Once into Trapping/ Grappling Zone, it is imperative that we use our skills to end the situation quickly and effectively. We will do this by using some of our strongest tools to accomplish this mission, which is to take out the opponent or attacker.

- ✓ **Punches**
- ✓ **Heel Palms**
- ✓ **Elbows**
- ✓ **Head butts**
- ✓ **Knees**

Most fights will end up in a grappling situation, as soon as the practitioner realizes that he can no longer be effective in the Kicking or the Boxing Zones. They will do the next most natural thing, which is to close the gap and clinch the opponent so as not to take the shots that are coming in at him.

If you look at professional boxing matches you will notice that the boxers go to a clinch quite regularly, but because this is frowned upon, they are separated by the referee. In the street there are no referees, so you must know that when an attacker or opponent goes for the clinch, you must know what tactics to use in order to avoid playing into your enemy's hands.

Like all zones that we are discussing, we want you to know how to defend against them, as well as know how to exploit them when fighting someone within the specified zone.

Grappling techniques that can be used are many, and some of the tactics used from a grappling perspective are as follows:

- Arm & Wrist Locks
- Finger Locks
- Chokes
- Pressure Point & Nerve Strikes

This can be an effective zone when you know what you are trying to accomplish within this zone. By the same token, if you are engaged in combat with someone who is far bigger or stronger than you, you must be able to move decisively in order to take the big man out quickly. This takes a game plan, which we will outline for you in order for you to attack and defend within Trapping/Grappling Zone.

Realize that when in this zone you are at a very close range to your opponent and he can hit you and you can hit him. One of the secrets is knowing that no matter what is taking place within the fight, you will always have a line of attack open to strike into. There are 3 lines of attack:

1. **High Line (From the neck to the head)**
2. **Middle Line (From waist to the neck)**
3. **Low Line (From feet to the waist)**

EXAMPLES OF LINE FAMILIARIZATION

(1) High line & mid line are closed due to both fighters struggling with grappling and holding the head and torso, looking for position to strike. Use Low line striking to feet, groin, using stomps, scrapes, knees etc.

(2) Low line closed due to both fighters trying to take the other down to the ground. You can utilize both the mid-line or high-line destruction's to neutralize the opponent such as: Punches, elbows, **head-butts, heel palms, pressure point strikes etc.**

(3) Mid line is closed due to grappling with arms, trying to push and/or get an arm lock on your opponent. Utilize kicking to low line or head-butts to the high line.

These are just 3 examples of many, but give you an idea that a line is always open for attack, no matter how big the opponent is. ***This is critical and must be understood by you for you to be an effective fighter.***

Some of the counters are mentioned above, but there are others when confronted with this type of zone attack. The best way to counter someone entering Trapping/Grappling Zone is to counter attack with your own ferocious attack within that zone based on examples above.

> ✓ **Move in and out, and try to not to let them close in on you**
> ✓ **Maintain position and look to get a takedown and/or enter Ground-fighting Zone**

The moving in and out is a difficult strategy, unless you have a lot of space to work with, as the opponent will invariably close the gap at some point eventually. Again this is exactly the strategy that you want to employ, so that you can close the gap on him and dish out your weapon of choice. We will be going into the Ground-fighting Zone and this is one of the ways in which to counter the Trapping/Grappling exponent.

GROUNDFIGHTING ZONE

Ground-fighting Zone is a last ditch effort in a confrontation, unless you get the feeling that

1. You are more skilled on the ground than your attacker.
2. It is not a multiple attacker situation.

These two caveats are very important when dealing with a possible ground-fighting situation, because even if you are in an advantages position, if there's more than one attacker you could be in for a world of hurt. It's hard dealing with more than one person from the Ground fighting zone.

"Never go to the ground with multiple attackers, and always survey the situation so that you know how many attackers there are!"

Ground-fighters are some of the most dynamic fighters that are out there, as evidenced by the success of ground-fighting within several "No Holds Barred" competitions that are popular on TV today.

"Some statistics say that 90% of all real fights go to a clinch and then to go to the ground"

If you can get proficient on the ground, you will have an advantage that most attackers or opponents won't have, but again it can be a potentially lethal situation if you're not careful. There are several schools of thought within martial systems as to the purpose of ground-fighting as we teach a couple of different methodologies where ground-fighting is concerned and they are:

1. **Take the opponent down to put in different holds**
   a. Choke Outs
   b. Arm Locks or Breaks
   c. Leg & Ankle Locks

2. **Take them down into a favorable position with which you can strike (Full Mount or Side Mount)**

3. **Take them down to apply pressure and nerve strikes**

All things being equal within the realm of combative martial arts training, having ground-fighting experience and enough knowledge gives you a distinct advantage over most street attackers and in most cases other martial artists.

There are several key positions when looking at taking a fight to the ground, and to become proficient at them is important in utilizing these skills against a much bigger or stronger opponent. Ground-fighting is comprised of some attributes or skills that we need to look at more closely in order to become proficient on the ground.

Takedown Techniques

• **Sweeps/Buckles:** *This is a technique where you would literally sweep your opponent to the ground with your feet. Usually by hooking your foot or leg around the back of their leg and pulling your leg forward while you push their body back. A buckle would be where you are sweeping in a violent fashion from the front through the legs, buckling the leg and possible breaking it.*

• **Throws:** *You can throw the opponent down many different ways, some of which are hip throws (Judo throw), neck throws, body rolls or throws, head & elbow throws, and several others.*

• **Tackle or Double Leg Takedown:** *Used by wrestlers and others, is usually a charging type of technique where the opponent can be taken down by tackling them like in a football game. This is a very good technique, but like any technique it needs to be practiced.*

There are several concerns when the fight goes to the ground, and that is whether you are on the top or bottom position. We will utilize some techniques that will afford us an advantage with either the top or bottom position. There are positions of advantage from both the top and the bottom position, and it is imperative that you know the strengths of each position.

We will not go into detail within the confines of this course, but would recommend you seek out a competent instructor locally to teach you the intricacies of these skills, but you will get at least a cursory understanding of what to do when the action goes to the ground.

Learning a couple of strategies of what you will do if you end up on the ground on the top or bottom position is imperative, so that like any other technique, you are prepared to take the appropriate action when you end up either in a top or bottom controlling position.

Positions from the Ground

• **The Mount:** *The Mount is a dominant position from the top position, where you have the opponent on his back and you are mounting him with your legs straddling the chest area. From this position it is very hard to get out of from the bottom, and very easy to punch onto the opponent from the top position. Normally the opponent will turn over to his stomach to escape your punches, and then you can choke them from behind. You can also do various arm locks and apply various pressure point manipulations.*

• **The Guard:** *This is a defensive/offensive position that is done from your back with the opponent on top. This is the exact opposite of the mount, except you're on the bottom. Your legs will be wrapped around the opponents body, and you will try to keep him close to you so that he does not have the leverage to punch you. You must keep your legs wrapped otherwise they can achieve the mount on you and then you will be in a world of trouble. From The Guard you can get many good arm locks, chokes, and some very dynamic, but vary rarely taught pressure points to submit an opponent.*

There is more to ground-fighting than these points, but the key is you have some understanding of which positions can save you in a tight situation. Ground-fighting is a great equalizer and will give you the advantage when you confront someone that is bigger or stronger, but does not have ground-fighting experience.

"A good groundfighter will always defeat a martial artist that is good at punching and kicking, but has no groundfighting skills."

There are ways to defeat a grappler or ground-fighter, but unlike the other zones, to defeat a skilled ground-fighter you must learn what their game is and how they will exploit it to defeat you. No one is invincible, but you must practice tactics that will work when it comes to a grappling confrontation. The good news is that most people will not know any of this information, so you will most likely have the advantage. If you do look to counter a ground-fighter, you must:

- ✓ Be able to negate their takedown efforts through striking and kicking methods. Try to keep a safe distance as a grappler/groundfighter is only dangerous in close.

- ✓ Know the Advantages positions of the Mount or Guard so that you can maintain the superior position in order to control the opponent.

As you can see, the advantages are many for each zone of attack, but to be a complete fighter you must become skilled at each zone. This is an advantage that will separate you from the common thug on the street, or even most martial artists. We will go into specific drills and training methods to get you familiar with each zone and how you can become proficient at each.

Real Self-Defense Methodologies

What we want to deal with now are some of the core methods and tactics you can successfully use in order to defend yourselves in a violent confrontation. Self-defense is a needed in today's society, but how many of us are actually prepared in the event of a situation turning ugly?

Some of the things that we will discuss in this chapter may sound a little like overkill, but the fact is that in order to successfully defend ourselves, we must learn some strategies that will give us the advantage in any given instance of attack.

There are many different types of attacks, and we will cover some examples to understand the best methods to use in each specific situation. From no confrontation, to attacks & fights, the situations are never the same, but there are some keys to understanding what type of situation there is and what type of retaliation is needed. There is a big difference between getting into a "high volume discussion" with a friend or acquaintance or someone pulling a gun or knife on you in the street. We will also take a look at some of the statistics on violent crime and where they take place.

Where it happens	% of violent crimes (Rape, Robbery, Assualt)	% of Personal Larceny with Contact
On Street/Parking Lot	36%	28%
In or Near Home	26%	7%
In a Commercial Building	7%	22%
On Public Transportation	1%	15%
Inside a Restaurant/Bar	6%	12%
In a School	9%	4%
Friends/Neighbors House	8%	10%
Elsewhere	8%	10%
TOTAL	100%	100%

Source: U.S. Department of Justice, Bureau of Justice Statistics, Criminal Victimization in the U.S. 1985

This table of information gives you an idea of where most crimes are committed. Here are some Criminal Awareness Facts, and how they could impact your life.

1. Today you have a greater chance of being a victim of a violent crime than of being hurt in a traffic accident.
2. In one of five robberies, a firearm is discharged
3. Thirty-eight states are now under court order to release tens of thousands of prisoners.
4. Fifty-nine percent of all violent felons awaiting trial were released into our city streets.
5. Guns and knives are the most common weapons used in robberies.
6. A rapist's preferred weapon is the knife.
7. The majority of rapes are premeditated.
8. Nearly 50 percent of all rapes occur in the victim's own homes.
9. Approximately half of all violent crimes occur 5 miles or less from the victim's home.
10. Robberies are most likely to occur in the months of Aug & Dec.

(Source: U.S. Department of Justice, Bureau of Justice Statistics.)

We want to empower you, so that you will not become part of the statistics mentioned above. These are some of the realities of life, and even though we don't want to talk about it or really believe that it can happen to us, it is a fact that we need to come to grips with.

Knowing what can happen is like a wakeup call for those that have never been in or thought about what they would do during a violent attack on themselves or their loved ones. I heard a phrase years ago that has stuck with me today when it comes to what we want our outcomes to be.

"Become a Victor, not a Victim"

This little phrase lets you realize that you can defend yourself and that you are never helpless in a situation unless you decide not to take action. There are several steps to dealing with an attack or situation and we will cover them in detail. We will also take a look at some scenarios as well as some true life situations and how they played out in reality.

Awareness

Awareness is the skill or attribute to be able to perceive what is going on in your surrounding at all times.

Awareness is important because you need to know what is going on in your surroundings at all times. Some people walk around like they have their head in the sand, and then wonder how they got attacked. No matter where you are at, you need to assess where you are, what is going on, what kind of people (or characters) are hanging around, and any other pertinent information.

Muggers, Attackers & Rapists, are looking for an easy target, someone who is careless and comes across as a pushover or somebody easy to manipulate. You need to be bold and confident and carry yourself knowing that you can and will defend yourself. Why would an attacker want to try and accost you if you will fight back or scream, and potentially get him caught doing his crimes. We will go into some of the mental preparations in the next chapter, but this plays an important role in being able to eliminate yourself from some maniacs "hit list" to begin with.

When you are in a mall parking lot, do you notice what is going on around you? Can you perceive if danger is near? Are you prepared to take action, if action is called for? These are questions that you must be able to answer in the affirmative, as they are critical to you being aware of what's going on around you.

"The Key to Awareness is being able to remove yourself from a situation before it ever takes place."

Without strong awareness skills, even if you are a highly skilled fighter, you can lose the confrontation before it even starts. This is the single most important skill, to know what is going on in whatever environment you are in.

Training awareness is just as important as training in the physical realm. Using your awareness skill can save you many times from getting away from a harmful situation before it ever even gets to the confrontation stage. Some people like to take unnecessary risks, by going into unfamiliar neighborhoods or areas without thinking what the potential ramifications can be.

Here are some examples of some "Awareness Drills" that you can do wherever you go, just by using your daily routine or work schedule as a model.

EXAMPLE #1: *As you go through your normal everyday routine of life, start to really notice what is going on around you at all times. Notice what types of people are milling around. Notice what the traffic patterns are. Check and see how far you are away from the nearest person. If in a big city, as you walk down the street, check out all of the people not only walking towards you, but the people behind you, and also ones that may be just standing there. Start to feel the presence of that particular area, what does it feel like? A **point that you should really understand when doing this drill, never stare at someone in the eyes for an extended period of time. When you look into someone's eyes, you are sending mental energy to them and if it is the wrong type of person, you could be inviting danger!***

EXAMPLE#2: *Now we will take the awareness to the next level. As you go through your normal routine, and are checking out your surroundings, now start to imagine, what you would do if someone were to approach you and ask the time. What does this person look like? Do you get a strange feeling or one of comfort? What would you do if this escalates into a confrontation, and what was the person's intent from the beginning? Can you fight back? Will you fight back? Does he have a weapon? Do you have a weapon or an improvised weapon? You can do this type of drill while sitting in a chair, mentally visualizing what could happen and what you would do.*

Example #3: *Visualize your house. Using your bedroom is a good place to start. If you were to hear someone in your house in the middle of the night, what is the nearest weapon or improvised weapon you have? If someone was right next to you, what would be your next most available weapon? Maybe it is a lamp, or a book, maybe even a glass of water by the bedside.*

This drill allows you to mentally pre-play how you would react to an event before it ever happens. This is one of the keys to successful protection measures.

There are many other examples and scenarios that you can use, but this gives you the general idea of a "what if". When I go to New York City on business, I always do these types of drills to keep my awareness up. I always make a conscious habit of knowing what is going on in whatever environment I am in.

Awareness training is simple, yet most Karate schools never even emphasize it , and if they do they don't give you drills in which to train with. Remember that awareness is the first area you want to master in order to eliminate unwanted confrontations.

De-Escalation & Verbal Skills

The ability to diffuse or talk your way out of a confrontation or situation before it even starts.

In order to become fully capable to defend yourself, you must also become proficient at the verbal and de-escalation skills needed to get out of a harmful situation rather than letting it get to a physical confrontation.

Sometimes trying to reason with an attacker or someone that is bent on hurting you or a loved one, may be people one way to get out of a sticky situation. Realize that we must use verbal skills to get along with people every day, and this is no different. When it comes to avoiding trouble, sometimes you can talk your way out of trouble and sometimes you can't. But you must use every means at your disposal in order to achieve the results that you want. In de-escalating a situation you must:

A. Maintain a Non-Aggressive Demeanor

In the movie "Taxi Driver", Robert Deniro played the character Travis Bickel, and he was famous for saying the lines, "YOU LOOKIN AT ME?". This is great for the movies but has no place when trying to deal with a possible hostile situation or person.

A non-aggressive demeanor is a way in which you can remain calm even though a situation may be escalating. This means if someone were to come up to you and say, "YOU LOOKIN AT ME?" The proper response is not: you wouldn't look at him because he's too ugly; or that you weren't looking at him, but at his girlfriend; those replies might escalate, you'd do better off saying that you may have glanced his way, but you don't mean anything by it and that you're sorry.

This will defuse his initial emotional questioning and put him in more of a state of "Interpreted Control", which means for the time being he feels in charge, because he has perceived that you have backed down from him, and he will either continue the "inquisition" or he will leave you alone.

If his intent is to hurt you in some way you have set him up to your real capabilities as you have given him the perception that you are intimidated, but in reality you are the wolf in sheep's clothing! This is a very successful tactic that we call..........

B. Feinting Intimidation or Submission

A feint is a fake action, it is a false interpretation of the real thing. This is one of the "Secrets of Self-Defense" that are very rarely taught, as most martial arts instructors are macho and tough, and want to give the impression that they could never be afraid. They might even tell you to act tough in the face of aggression. To act the tough guy part, you had better be tough or you may be in for a big surprise!

Our art is the art of the surprise, it is sneaky, we cheat, we confuse, we'll fake out the opponent or attacker to our real skills. These are the methods that will pull you through a tough situation, and in most cases will also get you out of unnecessary situations or confrontations.

You really have to know when to stop being Mr. Nice Guy and when to move into action. You can win the majority of altercations, if you use the methods described here. Fighting is much more than just the physical, and knowing this gives you the advantage over most attackers.

Taking Action

This is the attribute to be able to know when it is time to fight, and having the mental toughness to do it in a totally controlled and prepared fashion.

We must know when to cross the line and move into the next phase of action. We must know within our heart that when the time comes, we can go from being calm and relaxed to going to the point of no return.

Which in this case is crossing the line from passive non-aggression to deliberate violent action, with only one thing in mind, and that is to dispose of our opponent in the most efficient and effective means possible, even if it requires deadly force.

EXAMPLE: *You are at restaurant or bar, and someone thinks you are eyeballing them or their girlfriend. They approach you trying to start trouble (you get the feeling they are looking for trouble). Your reaction should be:*

Submissive Posture*: Hands held up, and you telling this person that you don't want any trouble. You are standing in a side stance, which hides all of your "centerline" targets, hands raised submissively (as if to say "I give up"). This is an illusion to the antagonist as you are in reality prepared and ready for action. With your hands up, they are ready to block or strike. Your body is turned so that vital targets are turned and not available to attack.*

- You try and calm the person down by using a low and relaxed tone of voice, letting them know you want no trouble.
- They persist, and start to touch you or shove you. My rule is, if someone touches me it's time to go to work! The key here is that you have to have the ability to go from relaxed to totally berserk in a matter of seconds, and you need to know what kind of attack you are going to use.
- Quick "Snap Kicks" to the groin, shin or knee work very well as opening techniques.
- Close the gap and use a flurry of knees, elbows and head-butts.
- Close the gap and take the person down to the ground and either mount them or choke them out.

In this type of scenario it is important that when you decide to strike that you are totally committing to win the fight, and that you won't be done until your opponent has fully submitted or is incapacitated (knocked out, choked out, broken limb, etc.) We also want to use a concept that isn't taught often, but is critical when getting into an altercation. That concept is:

Closing Shop

Means that when you have finished the altercation you make sure that the opponent is not going to get up and attack you again or one or more of his buddies will do the same.

Closing Shop is important in any scenario as you must survey what has just gone on to make sure you're not going to get jumped after you have disposed of the opponent. This also means making sure you're not followed or leaving yourself exposed to future entanglements. Closing Shop could mean getting away from a scene to avoid legal ramifications as well.

Handling High Stress Situations

You might be thinking haven't we already been talking about high stress situations? Well we have, but there is a difference between a fight at a bar and someone that is trying to mug you with a weapon.

Every situation has its concerns, and what we want to address next is the high intensity of robbery, rape, carjacking, and other extremely violent situations. Every person is susceptible to being defeated and we will utilize every strategy that we have at our disposal. Here are some areas to exploit on an armed attacker:

The Five (5) Weaknesses

The 5 Weaknesses are emotions that we can exploit on our attacker to manipulate him to our advantage

(1)   **Anger:** *This emotion can be exploited in a way that makes the attacker so mad, that he lets down his guard for even a brief moment giving you a small entrance into getting out of the situation. One precaution is that with anger, you can make the attacker even more violent, reversing the situation to their favor and putting you in an even worse situation than before.*

(2)   **Fear:** *The attacker that is showing fear, could be the most dangerous of them all, as they are nervous and might do anything, including murder in order to not get caught. Someone that is fearful can be exploited by giving them the feeling that they might get caught, causing them to flee. We will cover more of how to mentally deal with this in the next chapter.*

(3)   **Lust:** *The rapist has lust on their mind, and a woman could ease the attacker by feinting interest in the man, only to react by pulling violently on his testicles, gouging the eyes, slamming the throat, waiting for the right moment.*

(4)   **Greed:** *The attacker or mugger only motivated by greed is easy in that all you have to do is give them some money and they may leave. This is also a way to trick them by saying that you have more money in your back pocket or your shoe, thus drawing their attention to their own greed, not your aggressive tactics if need be.*

(5)   **Sympathy:** *Feel sorry for your assailant and he will drop his guard if this is his weakness. Maybe he feels sorry for you and you can exploit that as well.*

This gives you some idea of some weaknesses that we as humans have. We all have some, if not all of those. Your common street thug may have more than one that you can discern. These things can be exploited, but we want to make you aware that every situation is different and that these types of events are unpredictable as are the attackers themselves.

You can always be deceptive and give off a false impression to those that might cause us harm. Don't underestimate how effective these type techniques can work.

"Being sneaky, deceptive and/or giving a false illusion to an attacker is the key to successful self-defense and must be internalized, and ready to be used if need be".

EXAMPLE: *You are in an unfamiliar neighborhood and approached by a rather scary looking individual. He approaches you, grabs you by the back of your neck, and demands your wallet.*

> • *You put yourself in a submissive mode like before, with a scared look in your eyes. Remember you are the wolf in sheep's clothing, acting a part that he is unaware of. You agree to everything that he asks, with a scared tone, and asking that he please not hurt you, thus giving him false interpreted control. Set him at ease, so that if you need to attack, it will be a shock and that you will be able to do it in such a ferocious manner that you will succeed in getting out of the danger.*

> • *Comply and give him the wallet, hoping that is all he wants, but you are prepared for combat if need be. If all he wants is the wallet, give it to him, as your life is not worth your wallet. If you feel that he could hurt you anyway, that is when you must be looking for the opportune time to attack.*

Everything is a judgment call in the street, so it is necessary to understand what could happen, and what your options are. When you train at home, even if you don't have a partner, you can do specific mental exercises together with the physical training, which will give you an advantage over other martial arts practitioners.

In serious high stress situations, you want to be prepared to defend yourself and use every available resource that you have. This brings us to an area that can save you and give you an advantage in any given situation:

Improvised Weapons

Any object that can be used defend yourself in a combative situation.

Improvised Weapons can give you a needed advantage when you need it most. Remember when we discussed awareness, we talked about noticing what is going on in the environment that you are in. Being aware is knowing if there are any objects within that area that you could utilize at a moment's notice.

When I was a kid, and was with my mother in the city, I would always be thinking, what would happen if someone tried to attack us? I would look around on the ground and see if there was a stick, a bottle, piece of metal, anything that could be used. Maybe I was just a little paranoid, but I was reflecting back on this recently and was surprised that I remember thinking these very same things that we are talking about now, when I was younger and less skilled.

Wherever we are, we can find something that can act as an improvised weapon. **Common items that you can carry all of the time makes for a great improvised weapon, such as a pen, a comb, an attachment to your key chain, or even money you throw into someone's face as a diversion tactic.**

Improvised weapons can be the thing that saves your life in the real world. Very few are taught the lethal aspects of everyday items that we carry. I really like the idea of ballpoint pens, as they are very easy to carry and when used right can blind an attacker, as well as be used on nerve and pressure point areas.

We would also recommend any of the popular spray weapons such as mace or pepper spray, which can be a very good equalizer. Depending on how far you want to go with your self-protection arsenal you carry around with you, here are some items that we know some people carry with them at all times.

(1) Pepper Spray
(2) Pocket Knife
(3) Chain or Flexible Weapon
(4) Pen
(5) Collapsible Baton or Kubaton for Keychain

I know some people that carry one or more of these items, and keep them on their person at all times. It all depends on the type of environments you're in on a daily basis, and what your needs are.

To deal with the violent offender, it is always good to be prepared. Can you imagine the surprise to a would be attacker, when you pull out your pen and gauge it into their eyes, or throat. Again we are only as defenseless as we think we are. We all know that these things can be dangerous, but how many of us would consider them as mainstays in our self-defense arsenal.

Vital Targets

Places to attack that will render your attacker hurt and you in a control position.

There are many vital points on the body that can cause severe trauma to the body with only minimal striking. Knowing where to strike is every bit as important as how and when to strike. The goal here is to defeat the attacker in the shortest amount of time possible.

See the chart on the next page for some of the best vital targets to strike in a serious situation.

EYES	*Temporary or permanent blindness, shock, unconsciousness, severe pain, watering of the eyes*
TEMPLES	*Unconsciousness, severe pain, shock, concussion, coma, bone fracture, death*
NOSE	*Severe pain, temporary blindness, fracture, unconsciousness*
CHIN	*Severe pain, unconsciousness, whip lash of neck, broken jaw*
BACK OF NECK	*Broken neck, shock, complete paralysis, unconsciousness, coma, death*
THROAT	*Severe pain, blood drowning, suffocation, loss of breath, nausea, death*
SOLAR PLEXUS	*Air starvation, severe abdominal pain and cramping, temporary paralysis, nausea*
RIBS	*Severe pain, collapsed lung, shortness of breath, heart spasms, air starvation, death*
GROIN	*Severe pain, fracture to pubic bone, shock, loss of breath, nausea, vomiting, unconsciousness*
THIGHS	*Fracture of femur, immobility, severe pain*
KNEES	*Severe pain and swelling, torn cartilage and ligaments, immobility*
SHINS	*Sever pain, possible fracture, immobility*
FINGERS	*Severe pain, fracture, dislocation, immobility of joint*
INSTEP/TOES	*Severe pain, possible fracture, immobility*

These are some of the many targets that can be struck to get the desired results from the hits. When teaching people personally, I usually will break it down to three main target areas to always concentrate on, which makes you think of those three rather than the 15 on the list above. Simplicity is a "Secret of Self-Defense", and what we try to do is make our methods easy for anyone to learn even if they don't have a background in the martial arts.

The Three Main Targets to Focus On Are:

- Eyes
- Throat
- Groin

These are the three main vital targets that you want to have in the back of your mind whenever you are training or going through different scenario training drills. The above chart shows you the capacity of the damage that can be done to the human body with the hands or feet. You should study all attack points and learn how to hit them.

These three vital targets can be deadly, and at the least very debilitating. You must know where you are going to strike someone, so that there is no guess-work as to where to go when you are in a difficult situation.

REAL LIFE, EXAMPLE: *I have a friend, whose father at one time owned a transmission shop in one of the worst sections of Queens, NY. It was not uncommon for people to not want to pay their bill when they saw what the price was. Now some of these individuals were not the most upstanding citizens, and would request their vehicle back without paying the bill. My friend's father (who is at 5'9, 170lbs, and 57 years old) would not be intimidated by some of these characters (for lack of a better name) and would tell them that when they pay the bill, they get the vehicle. Of course some of these patrons were quite a bit bigger and a lot younger than him, and would start trouble when told this.*

My friend said that if the verbal discussions got hot and his dad felt that it was going to come to blows, he would move into action. My friend told me that his dad would do the same thing every time someone got in his face, and that was:

1) Kick or knee them in the groin
2) Mount them and finish them off
3) Have them thrown off the premises

This is what I refer to as:

"Quick, deliberate action to a specified target"

My friends father was not a martial artist, he did not practice these techniques in a training hall or dojo, but he had the practical "street" experiences, and knew exactly what type of specific action he would take when the occasion called for it. This is the type of mentality and ability that creates specific techniques or tactics that you can call your own.

Handling Armed Attackers

What do you do if the attacker or opponent is armed with a gun, knife, club or other type of weapon? The reason people carry weapons is either for protection or for using them to harm or manipulate others. An armed attacker is the most dangerous type for obvious reasons, and can cause the greatest amount of stress to the person being attacked.

We want to now cover some of the methods that we can use to protect and defend ourselves against the armed attacker. Entire books have been written about defending against weapons, so this will be more of an overview of some do's and don'ts when it comes to weapon attacks.

I. <u>Edged Weapons</u>

Edged Weapons such as knives or other sharp devices can be a very real threat in a self-defense situation, and must be treated with extreme caution. We can't tell you how many times we've seen articles, books or videos that depict the most unrealistic knife defenses imaginable. We've seen knife disarms with the defender plucking the knife out of thin air. This is not only ridiculous, but irresponsible on the part of the martial arts instructor showing this type of near impossible technique to pull off.

When it comes to someone with an edged weapon or knife, you must show respect to the weapon being used, even if the person using it is not skilled with a knife. With a knife an unintentional strike can be as dangerous as an intentional strike.

We believe that in order to successfully deal with the knife, you should first know a little about the weapon from an offensive standpoint and know all of the knives capabilities. As you could see from some of the statistics earlier in the chapter, a knife is 2nd most used weapon in confrontations next to a gun, and is used most often in a rape situation. It is up to you whether you carry a knife when you're going into neighborhoods that you're unfamiliar with, as this is a judgment call and all of the potential hazards, as well as the legal ramifications, should be considered before carrying ant type of a concealed knife.

A. Offensive Knife Strategies

If you were attacked by a knife wielding attacker, and you had a knife of your own, these are some methods that you could deploy, when the confrontation is knife on knife.

• **De-fang the Snake:** *De-fanging the snake is the terminology that we use to fight with a knife. It's main concept is that by slashing or cutting at the knife hand of the attacker, you can force him to release his knife due to wounds on his arm, thus giving you the opportunity to take the knife's (fangs of the snake) threat away.*
• **Cut and Thrust:** *The correct methods for offensive knife fighting is being able to first cut the arms, legs or hand areas, then proceed to the thrusting of the knife into the bodies vital areas.*

It must be pointed out that the above techniques are dangerous life-threatening and life taking techniques and should only be used in the most serious of conditions. You must also be aware of the legal responsibilities of injuring or killing someone even in a self-defense situation.

Offensive knife tactics are important to know, so that you can perceive better what is expected from a knife-wielding attacker.

B. Defensive Knife Strategies

Knowing what to do and what not to do is paramount when you are dealing with a knife-wielding attacker. When it comes to fighting, strategy plays an important role in determining what plan of action you are going to take. When it comes to dealing with a knife attack, it is important to realize the dangerous situation you are in. Knives cut so fast and so easy that you can be cut, bleeding, and taken out very quickly if you don't react quickly. Practice what to do before it happens, as you really do react in a real situation in the way you've been trained to react.

C. Distance Control

The most important factor in a knife confrontation is keeping a safe distance from the knife. The knife, unlike a gun can only hurt you in close proximities. The chances of being hurt even if the knife is thrown, is slim unless your attacker is proficient at throwing knives, and most street attackers won't be. This means unless you are backed in a corner, try and run away to avoid a confrontation of this type. Fight back in these type situations only when necessary.

"The worst thing you could do is try and disarm or take the knife away from the attacker, based on an unrealistic notion gathered from other martial arts sources, TV or movies".

D. Improvised Tactics

If you must face a knife wielding attacker try to keep your distance. If you are wearing a jacket, sweat shirt, or other clothing that can be taken off, use the clothing by using it as a covering on the arm to protect yourself, while trying to avoid being cut. Also, as we explained in the improvised weapons section, anything that you can use to "de-fang the snake" should be sought (pencil, stick, car antenna, etc.) that you can use to nerve strike the arms, so they release their weapon.

E. Controlling the Situation

These techniques are used as a last resort, as it is very dangerous to control the knife or knife hand of an assailant.

✓ **Nerve Strikes to release the weapon**
✓ **Control the knife hand & disarm**

These tactics are when you need to do something, and you feel that the situation is going to turn ugly if you don't react in an appropriate manner. The knife is dangerous as can be seen from the following example:

Real Life Example: *A couple of years ago two young men who worked in a video store in Bucks County, PA were killed by a knife wielding maniac who came into the store where they were working. I don't know all of the details, but it seemed by the reports that they tried to fight the attacker off. Their best defense would have been to run out of the store and put as much distance between them and the knife. This may or may not have worked, but* unless you know what you are doing in regards to defending a knife, you have no business trying to disarm the knife.

I really believe that when people see a movie with regards to the hero disarming the knife from the villain, they figure that they could do the same. This is totally unrealistic, and should never be looked at as a viable option. Even trained professional martial artists and military men know the danger of the knife and treat it with the respect it demands.

F. Training Drill

This is one way to prove the point on how dangerous a knife can be, even in the hand of an untrained person. We have taught these type drills for years, and it is one of the best ones that we have seen to date. What you do is have one person or persons act as an attacker and have another person act as the victim. The attacker(s) are given black "Magic Markers" or similar tools to use as a simulated knife. The defender will be wearing a white T-shirt. The object is for the defender to avoid being marked by the markers being held by the attacker(s). What you will find is that it is virtually impossible to be un-marked by the markers. So, if they were really using knife(s), you could be bleeding badly or worse from the cuts. These type drills can help prepare you for those worst case scenarios that can happen in life.

This drill shows you how easy it is to get cut, and how difficult it is to get away from the knife-wielding attacker. This should help you to realize that you should never take the knife lightly.

II.   Firearms

Firearms are the weapons of choice for most thugs, muggers, and any other lowlifes trying to take advantage of someone. The gun is the most feared weapon that can be pulled on an unsuspecting victim, and defending against one must be taken with the utmost precision and timing.

"We will give you some ideas on what you can do if attacked by a gun, but want to caution you that a gun is the most difficult weapon to defend against, and we do not recommend you trying to unless you feel there is no other alternative solution other than counterattacking."

Hopefully you will never have to use any of the strategies employed in this section, as this could be a life or death situation and the utmost care should be taken before even considering taking on a person with a gun.

A gun can go off just as easily accidentally as it could by intent, which is one of the many reasons why you don't want to take this lightly. Many people have been injured or killed by the accidental firing of guns even while cleaning them or showing them to a friend or family member. Since most attackers are usually nervous, afraid, or even intoxicated or on drugs, at the time, you can't rely on them to think or move in a rational manner, **so again please use the utmost caution with these concepts.**

A. Firearms Defense Tactics

When we discussed edged weapons, we stressed the importance of keeping a safe distance from the knife, so as to be unreachable from the weapon, with a gun we want to do the exact opposite which is to stay as close to the opponent as possible to control the weapon.

"When in a firearms situation, if you feel you have no other choice than to defend, you must get control of the weapon, so that it doesn't discharge at you".

If an attacker maintains a safe distance from you it will be harder for you to get control of the gun, thus limiting your attempts to get control of the weapon. When facing an attacker armed with a gun, you must use every possible technique or tactic that you have in your arsenal in order to get control of the situation. This means using all of your mental and visual skills in order to psyche out the attacker.

1. Try to manipulate the attacker into a vulnerable position
   - By using eyes as distracters- For instance, look over their shoulder to the right or left as if someone was standing behind them. When they look, make your move. Again, only use this if you feel there is no other recourse.
   - Using verbal skills with non-aggressive behavior

2. Always act very scared and fearful as a ploy to get them to drop their guard. Once an attacker's guard is dropped, it will be easier for you to try and get control of the weapon. We can't emphasize enough that you should only go for the gun if you feel that the person is probably going to use it on you regardless of the crime being committed.

"When going for the gun, always try and get the barrel facing away from you in case it discharges."

An important note is that there is much conflicting methods on how to handle a armed attacker situation, and some authorities say you should obey the attacker and give them what they want. I agree that my life is worth far more than a wallet or purse, but that in today's society, you have muggers that often times will murder the victim to eliminate any witnesses to the crime. It is this type of behavior that makes the non-retaliation route just as risky as trying to retaliate in my opinion. You can practice similar drills to knife training drills with guns using a wood or plastic prop.

Car-Jacking

Car-Jackings are happening all over the country and are very scary situations, and a lot of times the victims are being killed for their vehicles. Again criminals are more ruthless than ever before, so you must train yourself to be able to react quickly and deliberately. You should be aware of impending dangers and be able to avoid them altogether.

- ✓ Stay out of bad neighborhoods
- ✓ Don't stop for anyone & keep doors and windows locked
- ✓ Keep at least a car length and a half of distance when stopping for lights, so that you can get away if you need to
- ✓ If someone approaches, don't be afraid to just drive off

One of the keys to this type of attack or any other for that matter is to not be caught off guard. Even if someone approaches with a gun, immediately drive off. Even if they shoot, they will have a harder time hitting you in a moving vehicle than if you are sitting there at point blank range!

The Golden Rule on Muggings

Everything in self-defense is a judgment call, and you need to have rehearsed what you will do in the event of something like this happening. There are some things that you should never violate in regards to being in an attack situation and this goes especially for women or children and that is...

"Never under any circumstances should you ever get in a car or go with an attacker to another location."

We don't know the statistics here, but we know for a fact your chances of being harmed go up drastically if you give the attacker more control by going with them to another location. When you are in a situation where you could become a possible victim, you must put yourself in the most favorable position, so that you can get out of the situation.

You may have to run away from the attacker with a gun pointed at your back, but remember that someone firing a gun at a moving target is a lot harder to hit than one that's right next to them. The down side is that the attacker could in fact shoot you with a fatal blow while you are running, but it's far better than going somewhere with the attacker and being raped, tortured, and then killed!

"The Key to Self-Preservation is Constant Awareness"

There are many different scenarios that we could go through, and put you in different situations, but what you need to know is that you must be mentally prepared to deal with these types of situations, and that is what is going to be covered in the next chapter.

Rules for Winning Street-Fights

1. **Never Assume Anything:** Expect anything to happen and remember things that can go wrong, might go wrong.
2. **Never Fight Fair:** Rules are for sporting events and games. On the street you must do everything you can to survive.
3. **Do Whatever it Takes to Win:** Use all of your tools both mentally and physically.
4. **Be Ferocious:** You must be able to summon up your animal instinct to go from calm to deadly in a very short period of time.
5. **Capitalize on Your Attributes:** Use everything you have to your advantage. Speed, strength, height, weight, skill, etc.
6. **Be Able to Explode Into Action:** You must be able to go from zero to sixty in seconds flat. Turn on the turbo, go forward and keep moving forward. It takes practice.
7. **Take Advantage of Zone and Angle:** Fight in the zone that your opponent is the weakest in.
8. **Control the Fight:** Dictate how the fight goes, select the Zone, get to the right line and control the pace.
9. **Evaluate, Analyze, and Destroy:** Anticipate knowing your next move and that of your attacker.
10. **There are No Rules:** Do what it takes to survive.

Attributes of a Good Fighter

1. Ferocity & Extreme Aggression
2. Explosive Mobility & Balance
3. Sensitivity to the Opponent's Weaknesses
4. Focused Intent
5. Ability to Control Stress and Fear
6. Timing the Counter Attack Successfully
7. Being Relaxed Under Stressful Conditions
8. Visualizing Success
9. Being Bold, Confident & Determined
10. Ability to Generate Maximum Power
11. Strength
12. Flexibility
13. Reaction Speed
14. Muscular Endurance
15. High Pain Tolerance
16. Good Awareness
17. Making Quick Decisions
18. Comprehension of the Four Zones & Line and Angles of Attacks
19. Being Able to Take Action
20. Having a Killer Instinct When Needed

MENTAL COMBAT TACTICS

Mental training is without a doubt the most important ingredient in becoming a successful martial artist or self-defense practitioner. We have covered several ideas up until now that will have prepared you for more of the intricacies that will be described in this chapter. This is the training that separates you from 99% of all martial artists that never are introduced to the mental side of training.

Some think of mental training as the ability to break bricks or wood with one's hands or feet, or being able to do some other type of "mind over matter" feat. This is what most people understand the martial arts to be like. The practitioner will say that he is using his mental focus and control in order to be able to do the demonstration or parlor trick if you will. Unfortunately this really has very little to do with the concepts of mental combat tactics that you will be learning.

Mind Over Matter?

"Mind over matter is the ability to be able to bring the mind under control in a high stress situation."

This is our definition based on what we are trying to accomplish, which is teaching someone to be able to protect themselves and their loved ones from ANY type of harmful situation. This type of training or mindset takes the same if not more effort than the external or physical side of training. We can control our minds a lot better than most would think, but there are specific skills that need to be learned in order to achieve this state.

We will cover some simple meditations and exercises that can be done to make the mind much stronger, and prepared for any type of situation whether it be a self-defense, job related, relationship, or other encounter. When your mind set is strong the body can be stronger, as the mind really controls the body. These will be simple yet effective ways to increase your ability to control your mind in any given situation.

How to Control the Mind

One of the things that will prepare you for a self-defense situation is to use mental training drills to establish the mind set needed for a serious situation. This type of mental stimulation can be very beneficial to prepare you in the event of a confrontation.

The mind really is our primary weapon and as we get more into the **"Mental Fighting"** we can effectively prepare for the realism of combat.

"Mental Fighting is the ability to control and manipulate the opponent before actual contact is made"

How do you control someone before contact? The key is in the "Intent" that you use when faced with a situation. Have you ever noticed that when someone is angry or upset or happy when they are around you, that you can pick up on those feelings? Well the same is true of someone that is looking to be a predator. If they sense that you are not to be messed with, they often times will go find an easier victim. Can you tell when an animal is in that attack mode?

If you give off the vibes so to speak that you are like a caged animal, you can transfer that feeling to someone else. Sometimes it's that sense that just warns us not to proceed. This can be done with practice, and can be practiced for all types of situations, be they martial or otherwise.

Drills

This is a partner drill and can be done with just about anyone

1. Set in your mind an emotion, but don't let it show. For instance anger, fear, sorrow, happy etc, and see if your partner can pick up on your intent or your emotions without you visually showing that emotion.

2, Do this drill at random when you are at a store or some other public place where you can usually tell when someone is in a mood. Just be careful who you do this with, as you don't want to send an emotion to someone that could cause a fight, like anger or fear. Stick with the good emotions or intents when trying to change the emotions of someone you don't know.

These drills will take time to get down, but you will notice that as you practice you will get better and better at transferring your intent or emotions to others. As you start to get the ability to pick up intents, you will become much more intuitive in every area of your life. The mind can be trained just like the physical body, because our mind like our body responds to the stress and stimuli that we feed it.

By constant repetition you can train yourself to do just about anything. This is important in combative martial arts training, because you can put yourself into scenarios and situations and then work out how to solve the situation.

"Planning the mental side of a confrontation prepares you for the event like an athlete prepares for competition"

The concepts that we are trying to get across here is that you must prepare yourself for the possibility of a violent encounter so that you can be somewhat ready to take action.

The reason I say somewhat ready is because you're never really ready for combat, and it may come at a time when you are not in the mood, or sick, or with a date or family members, late at night and your tired, in an environment that you are unfamiliar and the list goes on and on. The mental preparation is the closest that you can come to the actual event without being there.

Sparring can help stimulate your physical responses, but does not adequately prepare you for the high stress situation. The best of both worlds is to hone your physical skills down and work on your mental attributes so that you are prepared for any situation at any time.

Next we will go into some mind programming tips that you can use so that you can be ready to go if the time calls for it. Remember that reality is just that, and that the more realistic you train and visualize, the more you will be prepared.

Mental Programming

Mental programming gives you some methods that you can use to give yourself an edge in a serious situation. There are many ways to do this, and we'll go into one that we have taught for years and works quite well.

Mental programming is sending thought impulses to the brain to cause it to do what you want it to do

You must have something that will trigger a response when you say it to yourself. We talk to ourselves all the time and need to make sure that when we do that, the talk is uplifting and positive. I learned a phrase when I first started training in the internal arts and still use it today. You can use this one or one like it to give you power and self assurance if and when you need it.

"I AM CALM, BUT DEADLY"

I was told to say this to myself when I was in a situation that might warrant being calm and also the willingness to attack if necessary. When we say "Deadly", this is a mind set, an inner feeling that lets you know that if things get a little funky you can retaliate with devastating force. This is a mindset that tells your body to relax no matter what the situation, but also to be prepared if it comes down to **"Go Time"**.

Learning to relax in the face of danger is not easy and must be continually trained so that you can act with deliberateness if need be. I will outline for you some methods to relax the body and mind, so that you will be more crystal and lucid in all situations.

You have probably received this special document as part of the Chi Power Training program. It contains excellent information on how to get and keep your body in a very relaxed state. You can contact Scientific Premium Company-USA at www.chipower.com for questions.

By doing this daily, you will start to integrate your mind and body, preparing you for when you will need to call on both. When you get good at relaxing down, you can do it almost anywhere and at anytime. By using specific terms while doing this exercise you will train your mind to act accordingly based on repetition and verbal triggers.

Workout Drills

We are going to go into some actual workouts that you can do to sharpen your self-defense and martial arts skills.

Mirror Drills

When doing home training, one of the best tools that you can have is a full length mirror. With a mirror you can check your progress and make sure you're doing right, a lot of the stances, blocks, punches, kicks, techniques and drills that you are learning. Use the mirror to see that you are doing each technique correctly. The mirror shows you what you are doing wrong and you can start to increase your abilities with the use of the mirror.

Face the mirror and practice all of your skills. Another good tool to use is a video camera if you have one, that way you can really see from all angles what you're doing right and wrong.

Practice your combos in the mirror. Here is a list of some possible ones:

- *Jab-Jab Cross-hook & uppercut*
- *Blocking with hands and feet*
- *Cross Kick Patterns*
- *Stepping Patterns*
- *Actual Techniques (Your Martial Arts Style)*

The list of possibilities is endless and you can make your own as you go along. The key is to analyze your movements in the mirror so you can dissect and see which ones need improvement.

Summary

We have provided information that we hope will help you in becoming more proficient with you own martial arts and self-defense skills. If you have any questions, you can contact us at www.chipower.com or at spcusa.support@gmail.com.

Part IV:

True Secrets of

Extreme Flexibility

By Scientific Premium Company-USA

Published by Velocity Group Publishing

PO Box 9516 Hamilton, NJ 08650

© Copyright 2009 All Rights Reserved

Introduction

In this report, we are going to assume that you already have some knowledge or a regular routine that involves stretching positions. If not, then just about any stretching book can provide you with the body positions required to stretch specific muscle groups. Since most visitors to this site are typically internal and external martial artists, we have found it redundant to provide and illustrate stretching postures.

This information is focused on the actual techniques and methods needed to achieve VERY HIGH LEVELS of FLEXIBILITY! Also, we will provide a guideline of how often you should stretch and what type of stretching you should do and specifically when you should do it. If your aim is to achieve the splits, Chinese or American style, then you should always stretch your neck muscles and calf muscles in all of your training routines. DO NOT neglect these areas, or you will never achieve your goal.

Dynamic Stretching

This type of stretching should be performed prior to actual training. Most people warm up with Static relaxed stretching before training or competition, which is completely WRONG! Relaxed stretching is best performed after training not before.

Dynamic Stretching trains and prepares the muscles to perform in a manner that is similar to the upcoming task. For example, a golfer should warm up by actually picking up a golf club and start swinging the club and twisting his hips just as he would as if he was going to hit a ball. He would start slowly at first gradually building momentum and increasing the range of motion to full performance.

A martial artist who is preparing to kick should perform, front stretch kicks, side stretch kicks and back stretch kicks. These are all done stiff legged for those who are unfamiliar with the technique or call them by a different name. Again start slowly at first, gradually building momentum and increasing the range of motion.

Next, you should begin kicking a heavy bag with all of the kicking techniques that you perform. Start with low kicks using a low level of power and gradually kick harder each time. Then continue with the same kick and raise the height requirement. Again, start with a low level of kicking power and gradually increase to a much harder kick.

Continue this process of gradually raising the minimum height requirement until you reach your current maximum performance level. Repeat this basic process with every type of kick you use in your style of martial arts training. Don't forget to include spinning kicks and jumping kicks if you are going to perform them in the upcoming event or class session.

You should NEVER perform any type of classical/traditional "warm up" stretching before class or competition. You must train your body to perform on demand. After one month of Dynamic Stretching, you will probably be able to kick at your prior maximum level cold, without any type of warm-up routine.

After all, if someone attacks you in a real life situation, they are not going to let you perform warm-up stretches before tangling with you. This type of workout also strengthens the individual muscle groups for the specific task at hand, which is extremely important for preventing injuries. This secret alone is worth its weight in gold. If this is the only thing you get out of the entire article, it is enough to improve your level of performance all by itself.

Relaxed Stretching

This is the type of stretching that most everyone is familiar with. The problem is that it is used incorrectly. Relaxed stretching should be performed after a workout or training session when class or competition has finished.

The reason relaxed stretching should NEVER be performed before training is because it will increase your range of motion, but it does nothing to strengthen the muscles used in the motion. This is exactly how you end up with muscle tears. The body's tendons are ready, but the muscles involved are just too weak for the required action.

You should never be in a hurry to perform this type of stretching, so plenty of time must be allotted in your schedule. It is important to stretch the muscles until they are slightly uncomfortable, and then PATIENTLY wait until the muscles RELAX and become comfortable in the current stretched position.

Once this occurs, you should then attempt to increase the stretch a little further so that the muscles are feeling a little uncomfortable again and then PATIENTLY wait while your body RELAXES into the new position. Deep slow rhythmic breathing helps greatly in this type of stretching. Try to breathe in the same rhythm as if you were trying to sleep. This tricks your nervous system into relaxation mode and helps the opposing muscles in a stretched position let go and relax.

Again, this type of stretching is best performed after training, when the body has heated up. Relaxed stretching can also be utilized while watching TV or listening to the radio, but you must be able to complete your routine several hours before you go to sleep. In other words, you do not want to go to bed immediately after a relaxed stretching workout.

Isometric Contraction Stretching (ICS)

This type of stretching should be done on days that you are not going to train. If you are going to train, it should be several hours later in the day. The objective of Isometric Contraction is to make the opposing muscle groups fatigued and/or much too tired to prevent a further progress in the stretch.

The procedure is to go into a stretched position that is still comfortable. In other words, it is easy. Then gradually flex and squeeze the muscles into a contraction. A good approach is to increase the muscle tension one breath at a time so that by the 4th or 5th breath, you are flexing at approximately 70% of a maximum effort. Now, take in a full maximum inhale and hold it in, while contracting your entire body.

Squeeze your fists, your toes, legs, torso, arms, everything. Hold this complete tension for a second or two and then breathe out "like a sigh of relief" and let your body go limp. Imagine you are like a wet noodle. Your stretch should automatically increase as the involved body parts relaxed when the tension was removed. Don't let yourself go too far too fast! An inch at a time is more than enough.

Keep repeating this procedure until you can no longer increase the range of motion in the stretch. Never breathe heavily or hyperventilate. Take deep full breaths and hold them in your lungs to compensate for the needed oxygen.

Never contract the muscles instantly. You should gradually increase the tension with each breath until you reach full contraction. This type of stretching also helps to strengthen the muscles due to isometric exercise. Make sure you really give your muscles a good workout by applying true effort to your flexing and muscular contractions. After a short while, you will be able to make your body feel "Rock Hard" whenever you want. This is really great stuff, if you like to spar or kickbox.

Acupressure Points

By applying pressure with the tips of your fingers or thumb to the specific muscle area that is feeling pain during a stretch, you can significantly reduce the pain allowing you to stretch further on the next effort. This technique is best utilized in your relaxed stretching routines.

For example, if you are trying to achieve the splits, then you should acupressure your groin area and the muscle areas that "feel the pain of the stretch" on a regular basis, at least 3 to 4 times per week.

Again, do not forget to stretch your NECK and Calf muscles! Apply the acupressure in the shape of a plus sign "+" to the areas that are uncomfortable. Breathe deeply and fully as if you were trying to fall asleep. Imagine that warm towels or heating pads are being applied to the painful areas of your body. This will also help the muscles to relax.

Training Schedule

You should try to stretch at least 3 to 4 times per week. However, try not to do more than two days in a row if possible. Two days on and one day off is a good schedule if you are really going to stretch frequently.

Do Not FORCE your progress! Your stretching routine should be designed so that most of your stretching workouts are comfortable and just a little more difficult than a flexibility maintenance session.

Twice per week, you should have a real go at it and try to reach new levels in your stretching. This allows your mind and body time to adjust to the increasing levels of flexibility. Always give yourself a day off after a really hard stretching workout.

If you organize your flexibility program around these scientifically proven and well-researched methods, your flexibility is certain to improve. Make sure that you take time to strengthen the muscles used in your specific activity to prevent unwanted injuries. Flexibility without proper muscular strength almost always leads to an injury.

Please review some of our other training articles in this regard. If you have an injury that you are trying to recover from, always consult your doctor prior to beginning any stretching or physical exercise program.

"BONUS" Stretching Tips

The secret of getting stretched out is in using your body's pressure points. The main reason people don't like to stretch is due to the pain involved. They try stretching out to their maximum and by the next day they are in so much pain that they give up. However, if you use the pressure points (also called acupressure) while you stretch and then again after, this will usually be enough so that you won't have the pain the next day. The pain is due to lack of blood- flow. Without good blood circulation, the area screams out to your brain that it is in pain.

When you use pressure points in the area of the pain, it causes the blood to start circulating again and takes the pain away. For example, if you ever push down on the middle of a water balloon you will see that the water is pushed in both directions. When you push on a pressure point, your blood is pushed in both directions. Pushing down on the pressure point causes the blood to flow through painful areas which are constricted. Be sure you read pages 3 and 4 of the Pressure Points booklet to learn how to use the pressure points.

Using pressure points is more effective than using a stretching machine. A stretching machine stretches your muscles unevenly, the maximum pull being in the middle of areas being stretched. For example, if you loop a rubber band over your index fingers and start pulling it apart) you'll find the area in the middle of the rubber band will really be stretched. If you told someone to try stretching only the middle part of the rubber band further, it probably wouldn't stretch much more. However, if you told them to stretch the area of the rubber band next to your index fingers they would be able to stretch it a lot more than the middle part of the band. A machine stretches the middle of the muscle, but not the part of the tendon where it attaches to your bone. If you want to get more flexible, you have to stretch all the tendon areas (tendons are the end parts of your muscles that attach your muscles to your bones). This is why pressing down all along your tendon areas will help you get more flexible.

If you hit a person on a pressure point which is located on the chart we provided, it will certainly hurt them. Try locating a pressure point on yourself and push down hard and you will see what we say is true. As with anything, it takes practice to become good at it. When most people get into a fight, they're just trying to make contact and are not specifically trying to hit someone in a pressure point area. Through practice you can learn to target those pressure point areas and it will make a difference. The lines on the chart indicate the upper layer of muscle structure. The larger dots on the chart mean the pressure point is closer to the skin and easier to reach. The smaller dots are located deeper and you usually have to go through a muscle or tendon group in order to reach it. You will find it is easier to reach some pressure points by pushing on them at an angle, which will allow you deeper penetration.

Before you start doing a maximum stretch workout, be sure you warm up your body. This helps you avoid injuries to your muscles and tendons and allows you greater flexibility. Start out with stretches which will loosen you up only, but not pushing it hard. Next, run in place, use an exercise bike, or take a hot shower, in order to get your body warm enough where you can start stretching to your maximum.

- To get into a splits position, you must train your body to do what your mind tells it. This is done by stretching regularly. It is also accomplished by teaching your body to stretch in the right way. You should try to relax as much as possible, taking long slow relaxing breaths, as you stretch. As you reach your maximum stretch position for a particular stretch, you need to hold the stretch for at least thirty seconds. This will allow your body to adjust to the new stretch level making it easier to reach the same level the next time you stretch. After holding the stretch for a minimum of thirty seconds (up to a maximum of 10 minutes) while being as relaxed as possible, you should tighten up and hold for 5-7 seconds, relax, then tighten again for 5-7 seconds.

Stretch every day, but stretch to your maximum no more than every other day. After stretching to your maximum, make sure you again work on all the sore areas of your body. Pushing on the sore area itself, and then to the areas around the sore area will help take the pain away. If you find that the pain is not going away, you will need to take a hot bath in Epsom Salt for at least 30 mins. For best results, make the water as hot as you can stand it.

If you have any problems, please write or call us when you can talk to an instructor.

www.ingramcontent.com/pod-product-compliance
Lightning Source LLC
Chambersburg PA
CBHW080427270326
41929CB00018B/3193